Kids Yoga
Suzie Cues

Alignment Cues for Children's Yoga

Rita Rainieri Polak, RCYT

ISBN-13:
978-1543014334

ISBN-10:
154301433X

DEDICATION and ACKNOWLEDGEMENTS

Suzie Cues is lovingly dedicated to my amazing husband Stephen.
You are resilience, perseverance, love, and strength.
Thank you for your courage to shine light on self-awareness and mindfulness.
Not only in our home, but also in every life you touch.

For my beautiful children Jack and Taylor,
who teach me about the world and myself every day
through innocence and wonderment.

This book embraces special dedication to my gracious and cherished parents,
Dr. and Mrs. Jack Rainieri.
The world is a better place because of the quality of your love.

This book salutes the incredible spirit of the teachers of the world,
including my sister Nancy.
She and her husband Rob embody the determination
and endurance to parent and teach through both challenge and triumph.

Thank you Arlene Mehlman, my yoga teacher in college
at the Fashion Institute of Technology.
You were the catalyst to my journey with yoga.

Thank you Judy Levin, E-RYT, RYT500, RCYT

Table of Contents

Sequence III

A Note From the Author

Foreword

There is contentment and joy associated with sharing knowledge and expertise.

As a practicing professional, I obtain satisfaction daily as I improve my patient's health and self esteem. My wife and I were especially pleased to witness our daughter discovering and sharing that same joy with the composition of this book.

Today, our children are inundated with digital data, which pulls them into visual and sound attractions of all kinds. This creates an urgent need for direction towards mindful practice that will allow them to focus their impressionable minds on their inner world, providing balance, and the ability to properly control impulses.

Neuroscientists have shown that the practice of yoga and mindfulness has an explicit impact on the brain's creation of gray matter and serotonin. It's understood that mindful practice immerses the brain's neurons with a supply of favorable chemicals that dramatically reduces life's stresses that can contribute to lower serotonin levels, depression, and anxiety.

We want our children to focus on life as it unfolds, understand how to properly cope with multiple daily distractions, and acquire resilience against challenges. All which will make them happier and better prepared for life.

What better gift can you give?

You may sometimes feel overwhelmed with the constant attention children require, however, give yourself permission to be mindful and present and to savor these precious moments with your children; their young years at home pass all too quickly.

Dr. Jack and Wilma Rainieri

Disclaimer

This book is for informational purposes only and is meant to enhance but not replace professional medical care, medical advice, or exercise.
All forms of movement pose some inherent risk.
The author advises readers to take full responsibility for their safety and the safety of students.
As with all exercise programs, proper discretion should be top of mind. Consult a healthcare professional before participating in the techniques described within this book's collection.

Introduction

Yoga for kids? Absolutely.
In yoga, our bodies help ground us in the present, as our awareness is directed to the changes happening within our bodies both physically and mentally. We are thinking less or not at all about the past or the future while engaged in yoga practice.
We simply bring our awareness to the present.

What does this book do?
Suzie Cues for Kids Yoga focuses children with the physical aspect of yoga while creating an imaginative mindful experience within yoga postures. The book is designed to focus kids' attention inward, while learning the most basic yoga alignment cues.
These cues are meant to guide children into the *approximate* shape of the posture, and guide kids yoga teachers into beginning to apply technique. This book invites you to weave play into yoga, using animal sounds, storytelling, and fun.

What are Suzie Cues?
Suzie and Jack are the characters you see in this book. They love the animals, pretending, and playing together. Suzie enjoys seeing Jack create the poses while she shares fun facts about each animal or pose. Suzie also has a lot of questions, whimsical ideas, and mindful suggestions that kids will enjoy thinking about. Teachers & parents can be inspired by and utilize Suzie's cues to create a dynamic and effective children's yoga class.

In this process, your students and children can begin to obtain the benefits of yoga and mindful thinking. While linking the physical techniques of breathing and movement with mindful practice, the variety of social, physical, and psychological benefits in almost unending:
Healthy habits of thought, the ability to tune out negativity, stronger life skills, strength, perseverance, optimism, drive, a spike in self-image, self-compassion, improved self-esteem, improved self-care, coping skills, resiliency, acceptance, memory improvement, mindful listening, empathy, compassion, emotion regulation, reducing aggression, experiencing peace, healthier eating habits, mindful eating, paying attention to the 5 senses.

We do not use our body to get into the pose …
We use the pose to get into our body.
-unknown

Sequence I

Kids Yoga
Suzie Cues

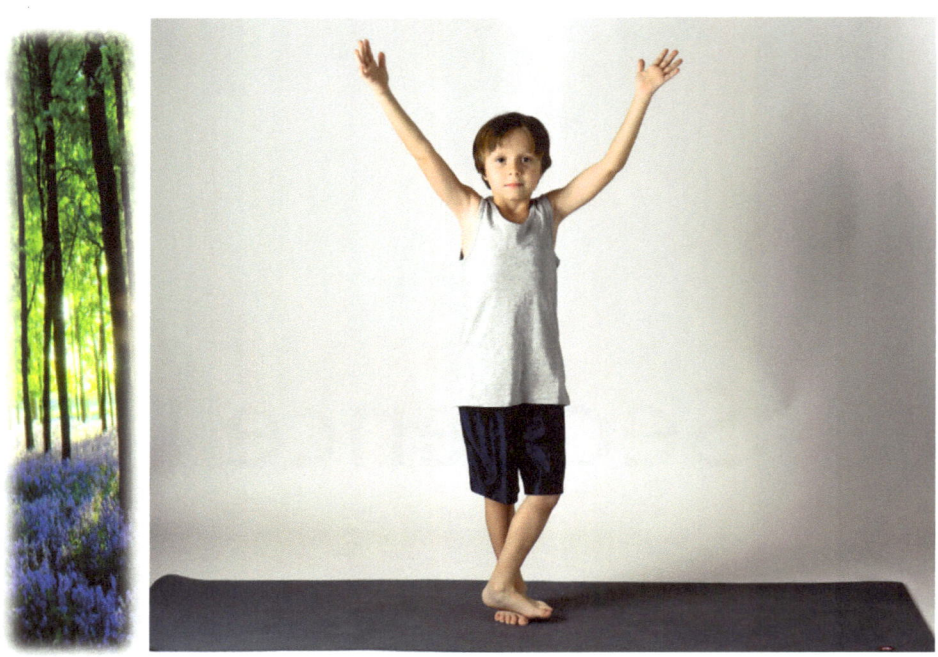

Tree

Vriksasana variation
(Vrik-SHAHS-anna)

Stand strait and tall.
Feel your feet grounded into the floor
as if you are the planted in the ground like the root of a tree.
Bring your heel onto the top of your opposite foot.
Grow your branches up tall.
Repeat using opposite foot.

☼ Improves posture, centers and balances.

"Trees have roots in the ground that give them water and vitamins.
They grow up tall and help produce oxygen with their leaves and branches.
Imagine what your Tree looks like!
Keep your legs firm like a Tree trunk
and maybe you can sway back and forth! Can you feel the breeze?"

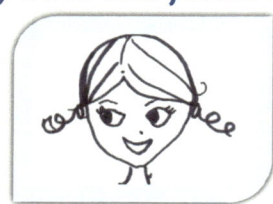

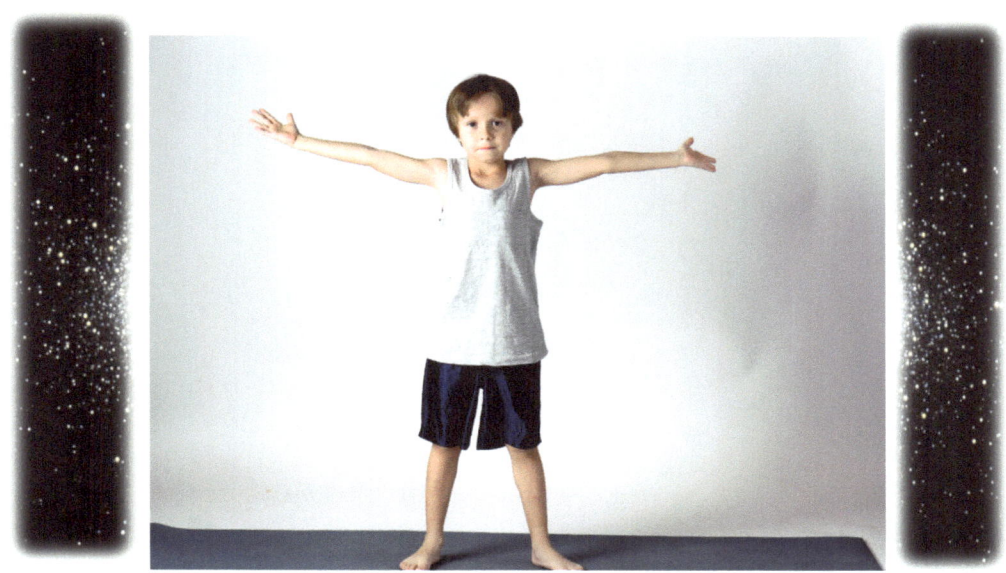

Star

Utthita Hasta Padasana / Extended Hands and Feet Pose variation
(Oo-TEET-uh HAWS-Tuh Pah-DAS-anna)

**Take a wide stance.
Make train tracks with your feet and root them into the ground.
Looking strait ahead, stretch through your sides
and reach arms out wide strait.
Stretch all the way through your fingertips.**

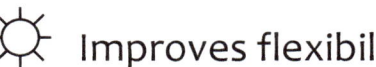 Improves flexibility and strength.

*"The nearest Star to our planet is the sun!
Stars form constellations in the sky.
Do you know what a constellation is??
Doesn't it feel great to stretch?
Make your Star blink: Jump your legs in and bring your arms to your sides.
Now, jump your legs wide and stretch your arms out again!
Breathe in, Breathe out, shine bright- you're a Star!!"*

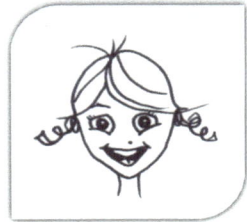

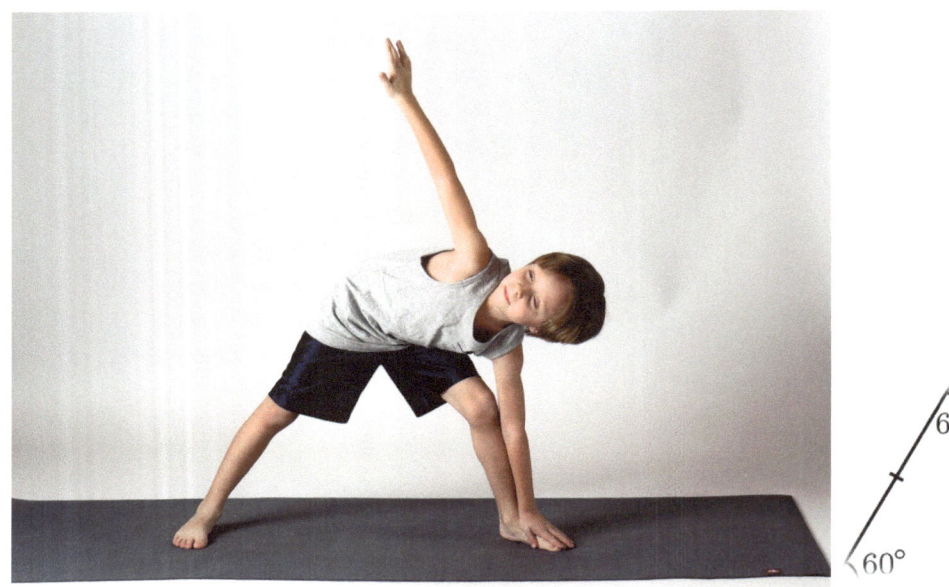

Triangle

Trikonasana / Triangle Pose variation

(Trik-cone-AHS-anna)

Take a wide stance or lightly jump feet apart.
Raise your arms strait out to sides, palms down.
Extend your body down to one foot with one arm.
Rest this hand on your shin, ankle, or floor.
The other arm extending toward the clouds.
Look up at your hand.
Repeat on other side.

☼ Stretches & stimulates abs, improves digestion.

"Triangles are polygons with 3 sides.
This pose forms an Equilateral Triangle with your legs.
Can you name some other shapes?
What is your favorite shape to draw?"

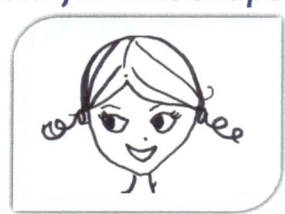

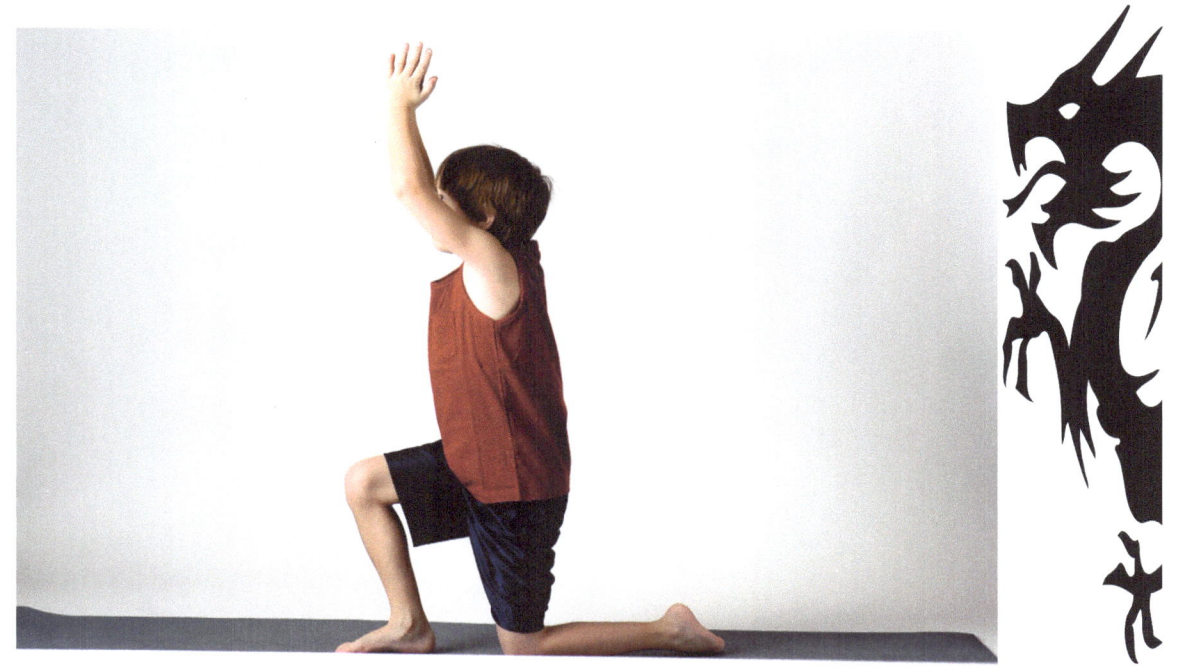

Dragon

Anjaneyasana variation

(AHN-jah-nay-AHS-uh-nuh)

**Lunge forward with 1 knee over ankle.
Lift both arms up strait pressing palms together above your head.
Lengthen your spine.
Repeat on other side.**

☼ Improves mental focus, strengthens knees, stretches.

*"Take a deep breath in, and breathe out fire!!
Are Dragons real or fiction???
Are you a magical dragon? A fierce Dragon?
Chinese Dragons are symbols of power, strength, and good luck!
Can you think of any stories or movies about Dragons?*

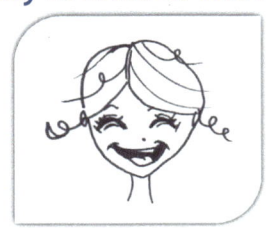

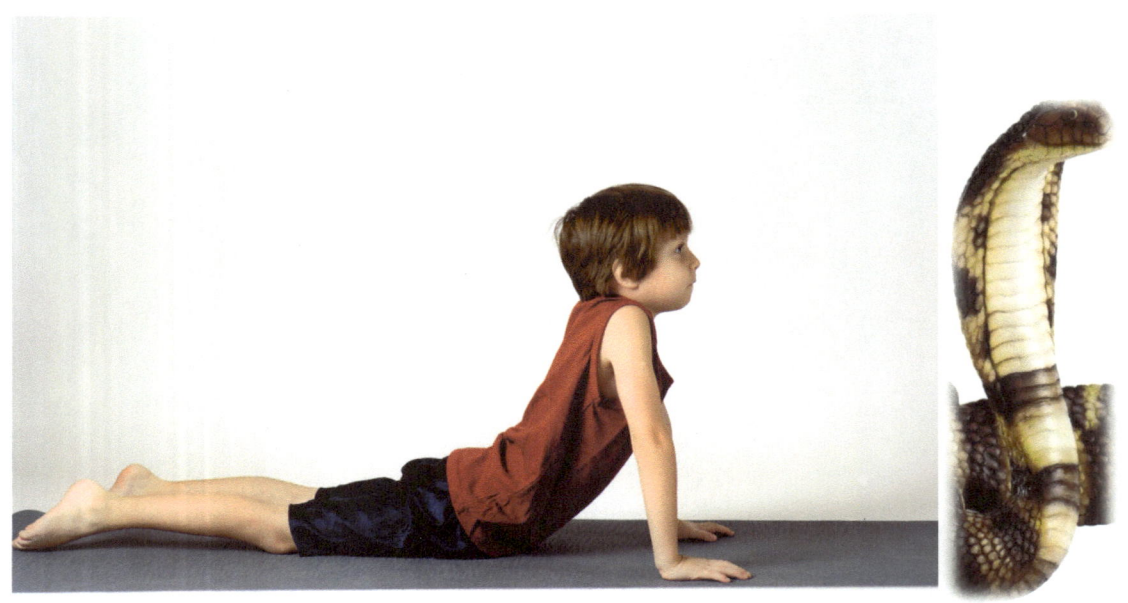

Cobra

Bhujangasana variation
(Boo-jang-GAHS-anna)

Lay on your belly.
High five the floor in front of you.
Lift through your arms and lift your chest off the floor.
Hands should be under your shoulders
and as you lift up into a snake.

☼ Increases circulation, tones back & buttocks.

"Give a hiss with your tongue!!
Did you know that Snakes smell with their tongues??
Snakes are covered in scales. Have you ever felt a Snake or a reptile's scales?
As you slowly raise your head and chest into Cobra pose,
imagine what it might feel like to be covered in scales!"

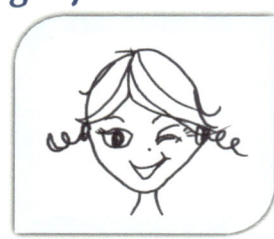

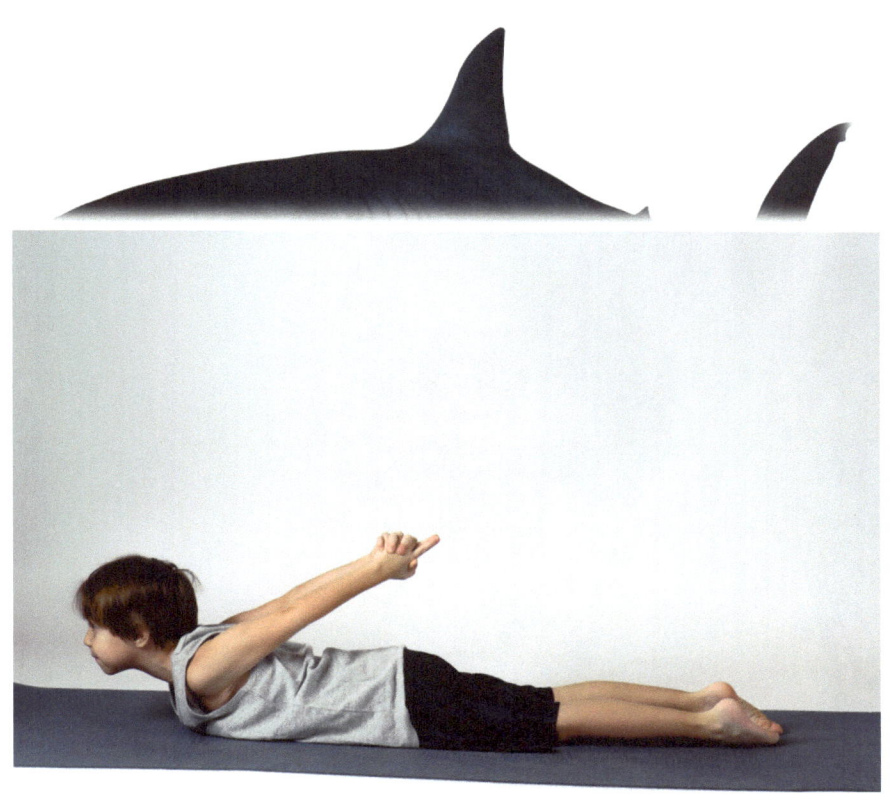

Shark

Salabhasana variation
(Sha-la-BAHS-anna)

**Lay on your belly face down with your big toes touching.
Palms together behind you creating a shark fin, arch your back.
If you can, lift up your feet.**

☼ Stretches shoulders, chest, & belly. Improves posture.

"What do you know about Sharks?
The largest fish in the world is called a Whale Shark!
Sharks depend on their senses to survive.
What are your senses? How many senses do we have?"

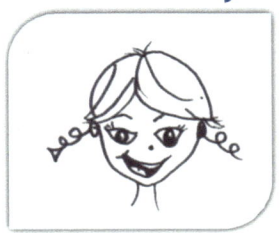

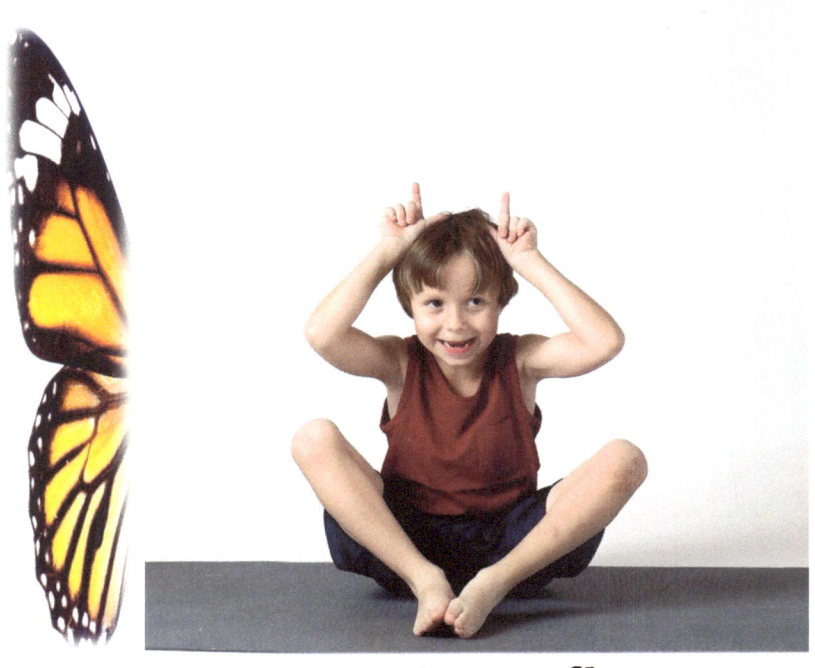

Butterfly

Baddha Konasana variation
(BAH-dah cone-AHS-anna)

**Starting seated up tall, feel secure in the ground like a plant.
Bring your feet together, touching your feet and toes together.
Hold your feet with your hands.**

☼ Calms. Relieves stress & stimulates digestive organs.

*"Maybe we can give our Butterflies antennae!
Butterflies are my FAVORITE! What color or pattern is your butterfly?
I like to chase butterflies when I see them!
They are beautiful to watch and very delicate."*

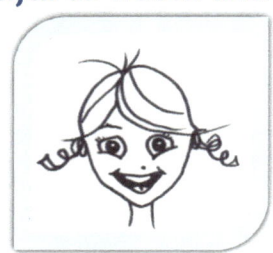

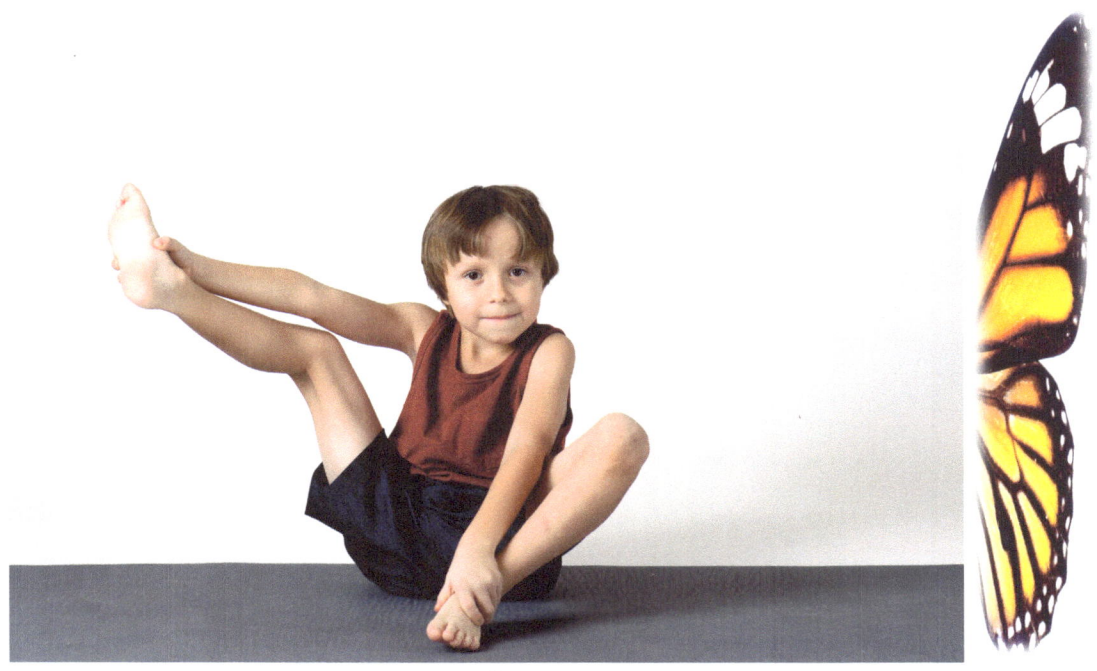

Butterfly Wings

Baddha Konasana variation
(BAH-dah cone-AHS-anna)

**While seated in Butterfly,
hold your feet with your hands.
To create wings stretch 1 leg or both legs open.**

☼ Opens the hips. Great stretch for inner thighs & knees.

*"Look at your beautiful Butterfly wings!
Try one at a time. Balance and stretch carefully.
Butterfly wings are very thin, almost web-like, and transparent.
What else describes your Butterfly features?"*

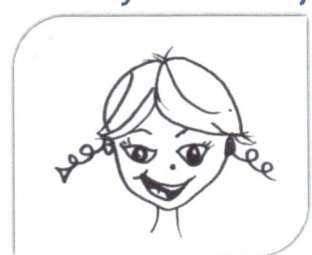

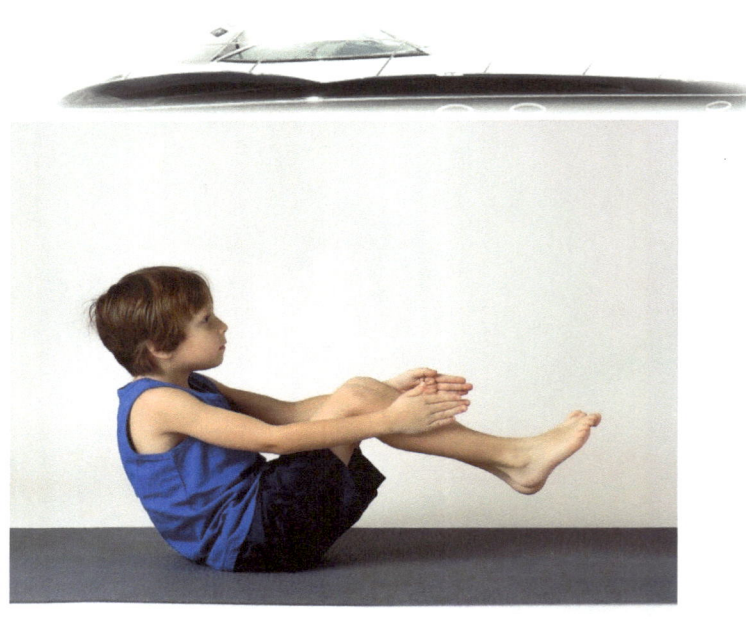

Boat

Paripurna Navasana variation
(Par-ee-POOR-nah   Nah-VAHS-anna)

Sit in center of mat.
Lift 1 foot first, then the other foot to create the front of the boat.
Lift both arms to create the sides of your boat.
Balance your boat using your tummy muscles.
Hold the outside of your knees if you need to.
Try to straighten your legs!

☼ Improves balance, strengthens spine, stimulates kidneys.

"Isn't it amazing how a boat balances
and floats on the surface of the water?
How does it feel to be in a boat? Do you like to go fast or slow?
Can you feel the mist of the water?!!"

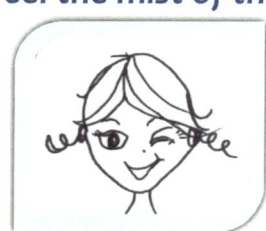

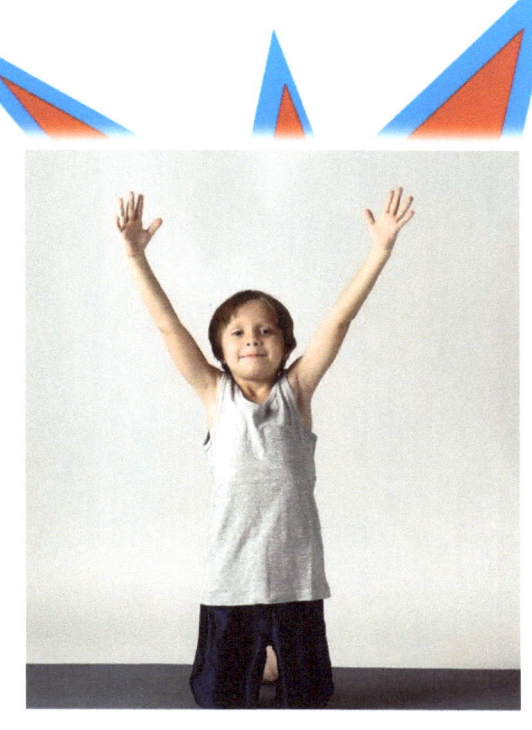

Superhero

Virasana variation

(Veer-AHS-anna)

**Kneel on the floor and rest your bottom on your feet.
Touch inner knees together.
Raise your arms strait up
and stretch your hands and fingers toward the clouds.**

 Increases flexibility in knees & thighs. Reduces tightness.

*"Who is your favorite Superhero? What is their special power?
What makes you special??
Let's all take a turn and talk about what makes us each special."*

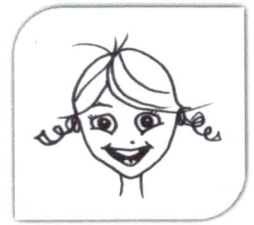

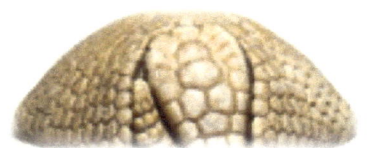

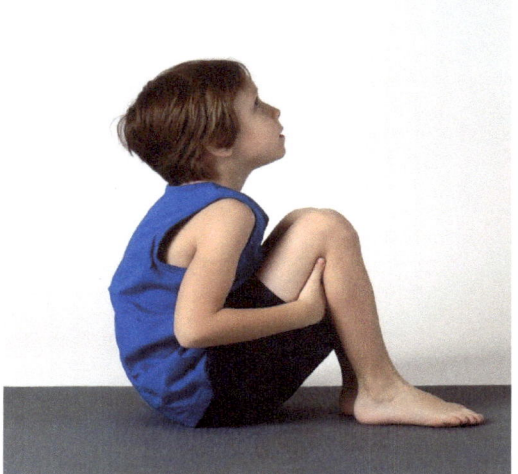

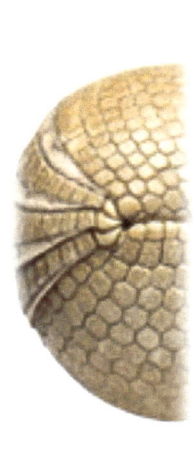

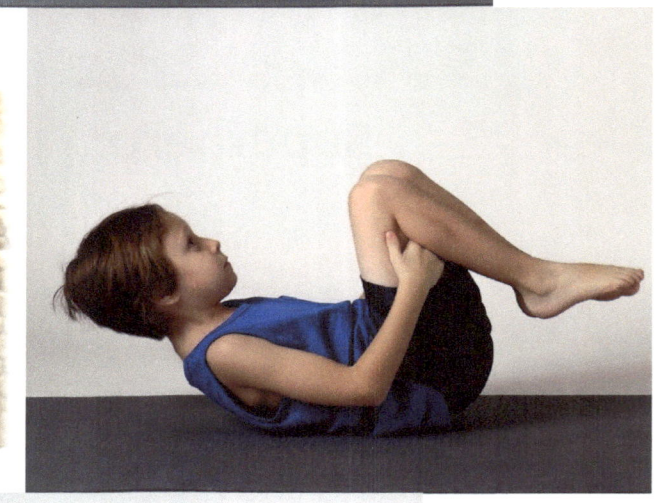

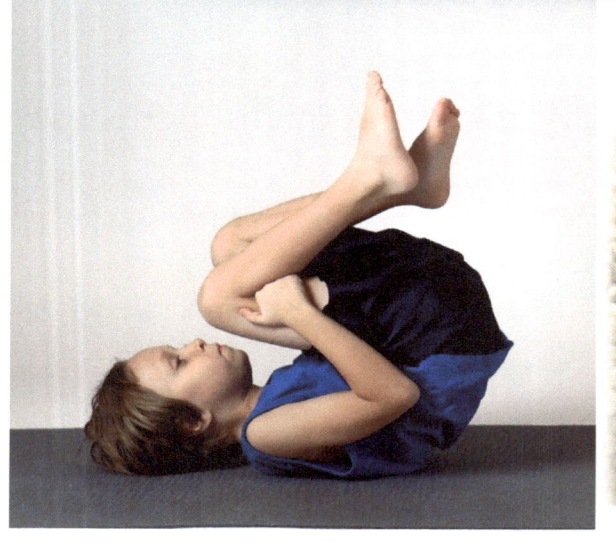

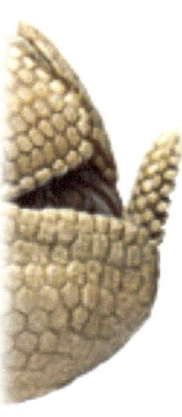

Armadillo

Jhulana Ludhakana (Rocking & Rolling) variation

(Jul-ah-na Lood-hak-ah-na)

**Sitting up with knees tucked,
slip your hands beneath your knees.
Tuck your chin down slightly.
Round your spine.
Gently roll back and then roll up to sit.
Repeat.**

☀ Great massage for the back, strengthens abdominals,
& kids love it!

*"Armadillo means, "little armored one".
These animals have armor-like skins!
Some Armadillo can roll themselves into a ball for disguise and protection!
Can you feel your spine as you roll?
Use your tummy muscles to balance as you roll up and down.
Pretend you are swinging in a rocking chair!
This pose just might be my favorite because it is so much fun!"*

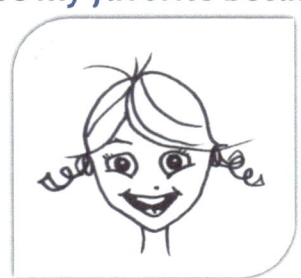

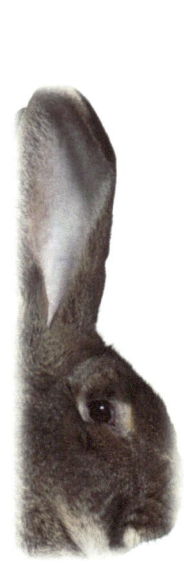
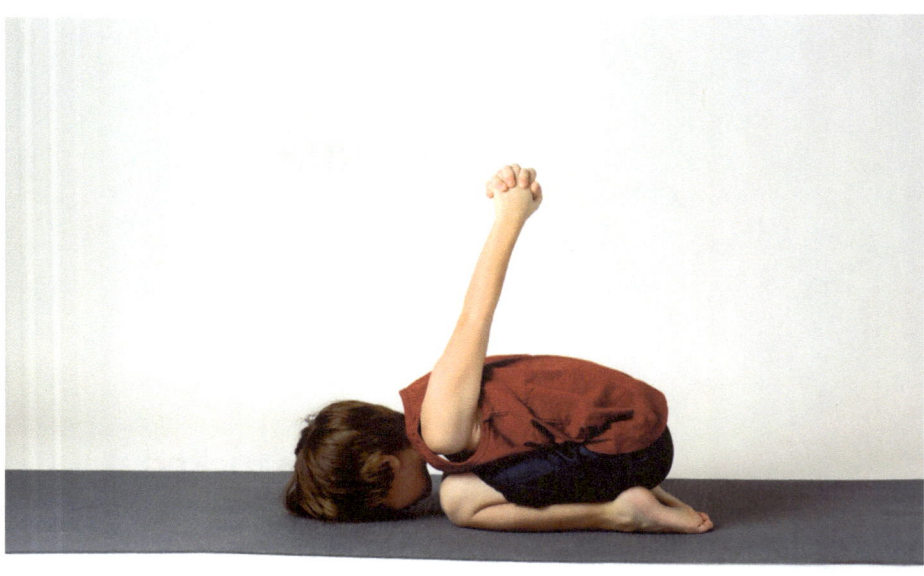

Bunny Rabbit

Balasana (Child's Pose) variation
(Bah-LAHS-anna)

Stand on your knees.
Lean forward and rest over your thighs.
Forehead gently touches the floor in front of your knees.
Clasp hands behind you.
Raise them toward the clouds to create bunny ears.

☀ Lengthens spine, relieves lower back pain, calms.

"Rabbits have long ears that average about 4 inches in length
and they have short fluffy tails
– but at birth they don't have any fur yet!!
And wow - did you know that Bunny Rabbits eat wild flowers??
Maybe you have a soft stuffed animal at home that feels like a bunny?
What does it feel like?"

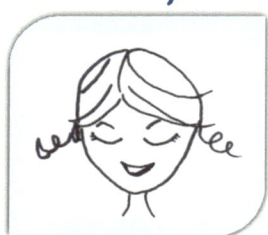

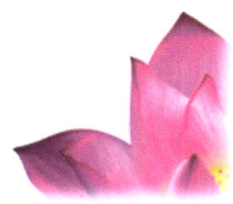

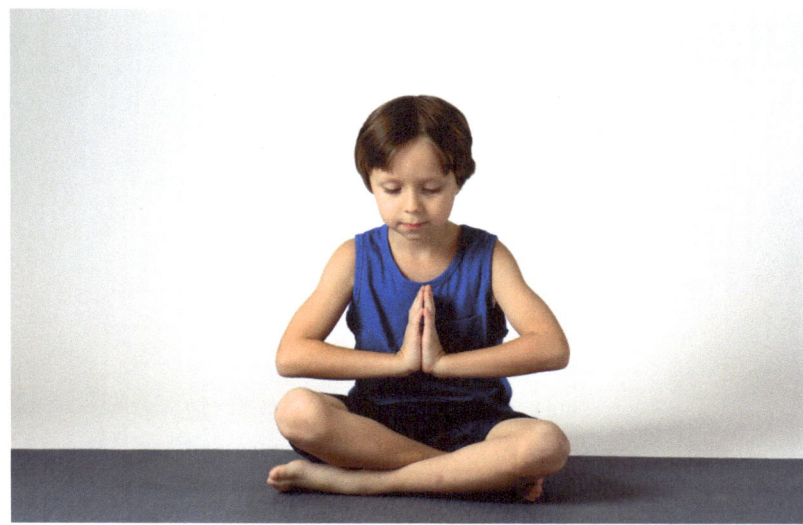

Lotus

Padmasana variation
(Pod-MAHS-anna)

**Sit like a pretzel.
Place your hands on your knees, palms facing up.
Then, lift hands to your heart, palms together.
Say Namaste.**
(Nuhm-uh-stey)
The light within me acknowledges the light within you

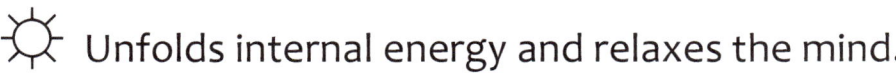 Unfolds internal energy and relaxes the mind.

*"A Lotus is a plant of the water lily family.
As you close your eyes, send love and kindness to yourself.
Then, send love and kindness to the ones you love.
Some other meanings of Namaste are:
The spirit within me bows to the spirit within you.
I greet that place where you and I are one."*

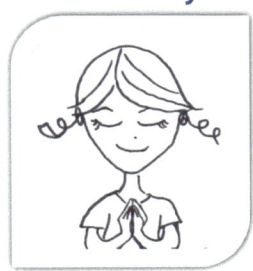

Sequence II

Kids Yoga
Suzie Cues

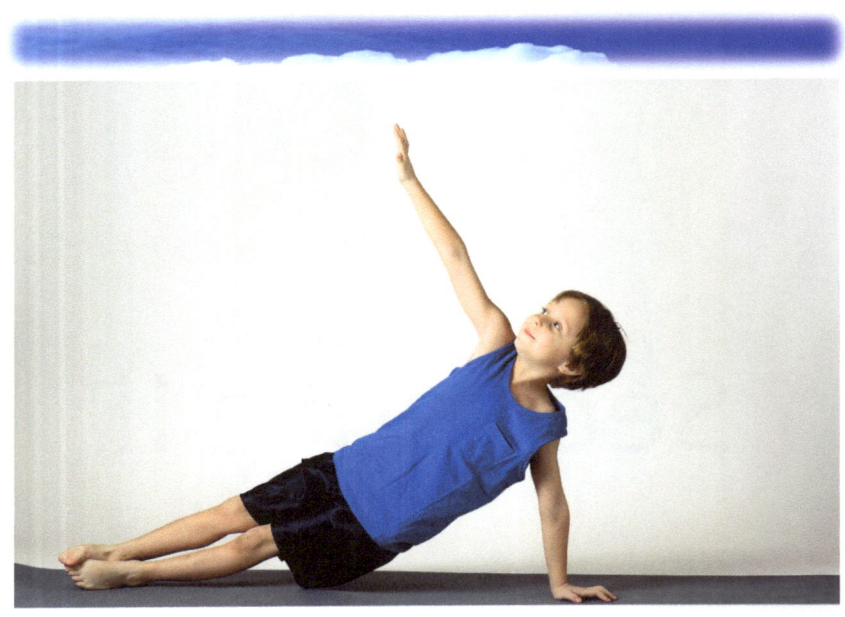

Airplane

Vasisthasana / Side Plank variation
(Vah-sish-TAHS-anna)

Kneel and take your arms out to the sides strait.
Press 1 arm into the floor.
Raise your other arm to touch the clouds.
Send your feet out to 1 side.
Lift up your body balancing on both feet.
Repeat on other side

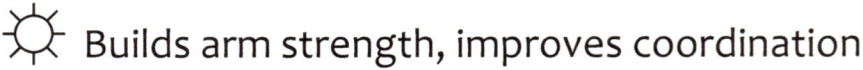 Builds arm strength, improves coordination.

"Have you ever traveled in an airplane?
What does an airplane sound like?
Look up at your top arm as you reach towards the sky!
Imagine where you will travel in your airplane, lifting up into the clouds!"

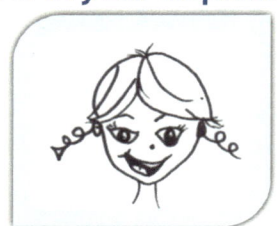

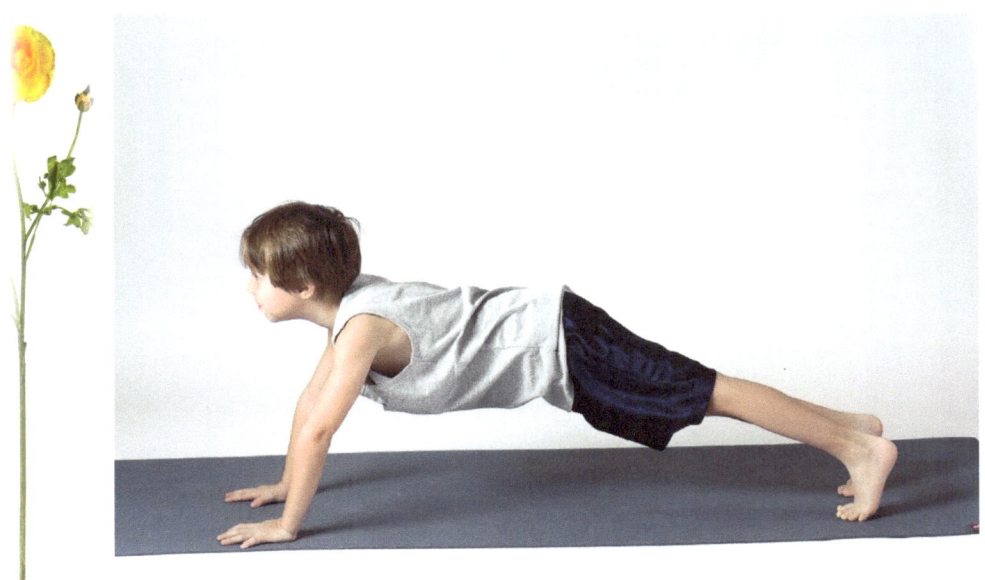

Stem

Kumbhakasana / Plank variation
(Koom-bahk-AHS-uh-nuh)

While kneeling, walk your arms forward.
High 5 the floor with hands underneath your shoulders.
Step 1 foot back and then the other foot.
Use the balls of your feet to balance.
Stay strong in your belly.

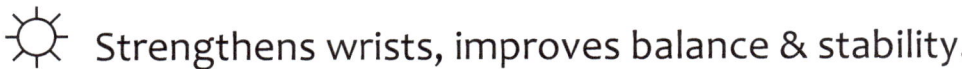 Strengthens wrists, improves balance & stability.

"Make your body strong and strait like a stem holding a flower.
Your head is like a beautiful flower.
Gaze at the front of your hands and pretend those are your leaves!
What kind of flower are you?
What color are you?

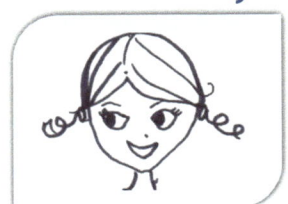

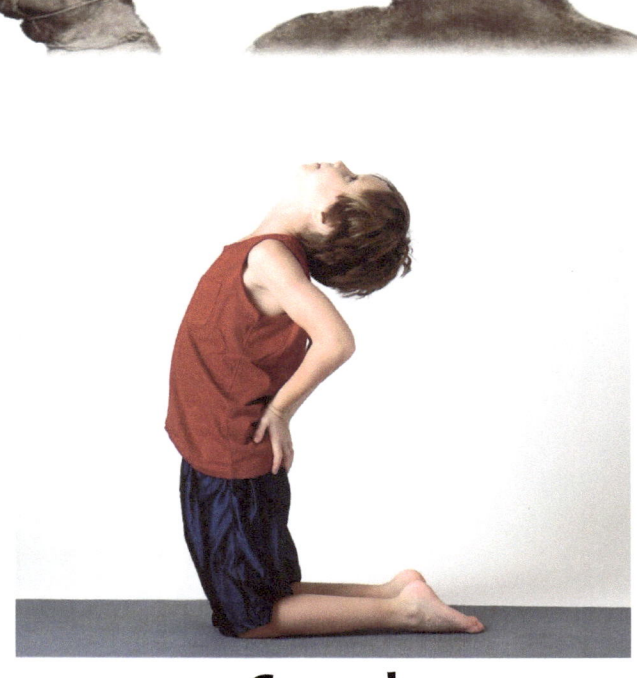

Camel

Ustrasana variation
(Oosh-TRAHS-anna)

**Kneel on the ground
and plant your feet and lower legs into the mat.
Place your hands on your lower back.
Lift your heart to the clouds as you look to the sky.**

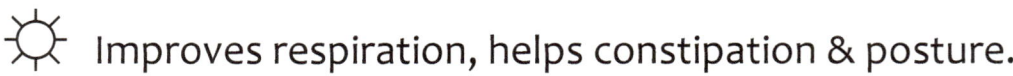 Improves respiration, helps constipation & posture.

*"Can you walk your hands down your back to touch your feet?
Did you know a Camel's hump is an energy source for them?
Camels have been called "the ships of the desert"
because of how helpful and valuable they can be.
What is something that is valuable to you?"*

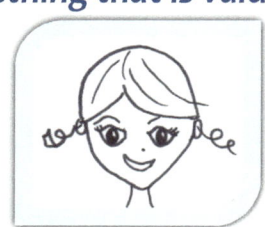

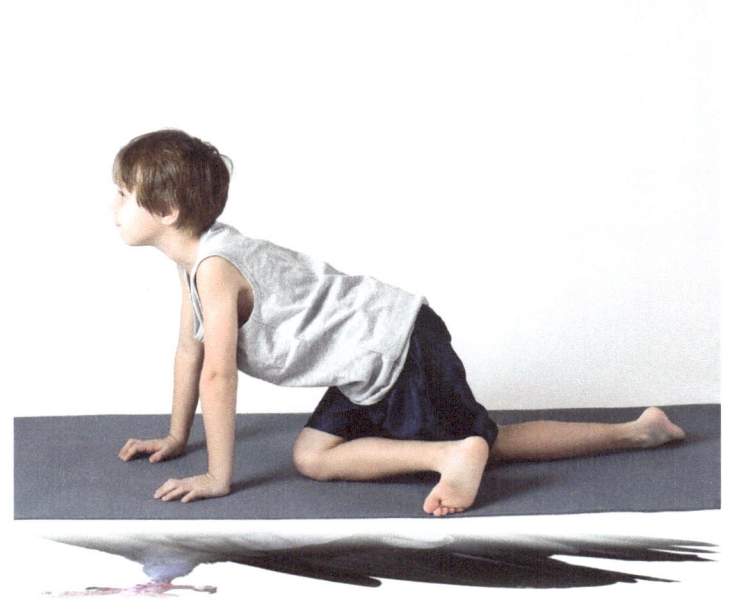

Pigeon

Eka Pada Rajakapotasana variation
(Aa-KAH pah-DAH rah-JAH-cop-poh-TAHS-anna)

**Seated in middle of mat, bend your front leg on the mat.
Stretch your other leg behind.
Place your hands in front of your front leg.
Grow your spine sitting tall.
Repeat on the other side.**

 Reduces congestion, increases flexibility.

*"Did you know that Pigeons see better when they bob their heads?
Some Pigeons are trained to recognize yellow and red lifejackets
so they can save lives at sea!
They are really quick and helpful.
Can you think of a time when you were being helpful?"*

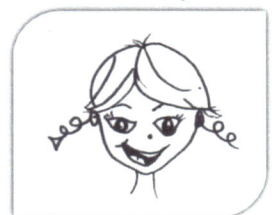

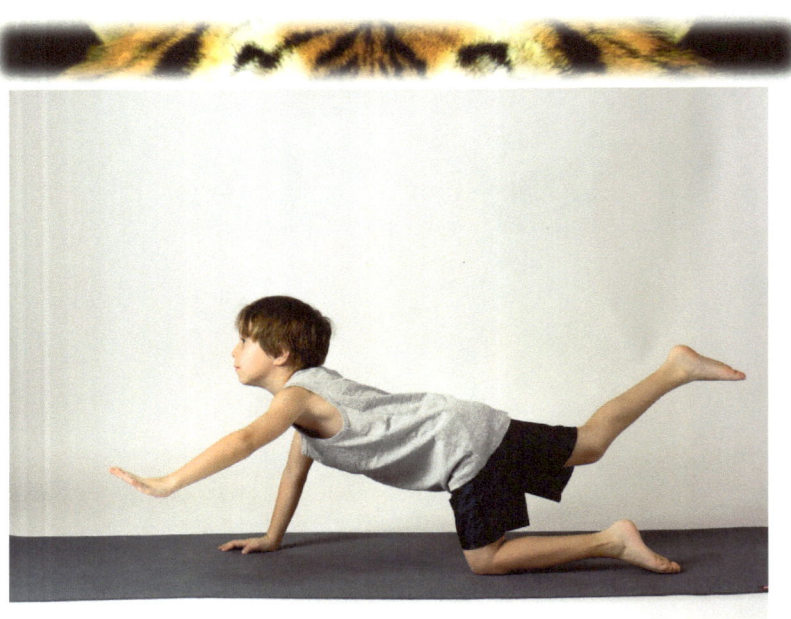

Tiger

Dandayamna Bharmanasana / Balancing table variation
(Dan-day-AHM-na   Bar-man-AHS-anna)

**Kneel on all 4s
Tuck your back feet under.
Spread fingers wide.
Stack wrist under shoulders. Bend slightly at elbows.
Reach forward with one arm.
Lift opposite leg back.
Repeat using opposite arm and leg.**

 Improves memory, focus, and core strength.

*"Tigers like water and cooling off in rivers.
But one of the COOLEST things about Tigers are the stripes on their coat!!
Orange, Black, and White... such a unique and wild pattern!!
What else do you think is something WILD in this world?"*

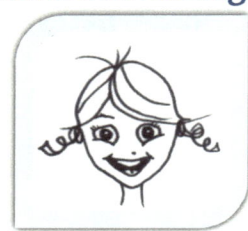

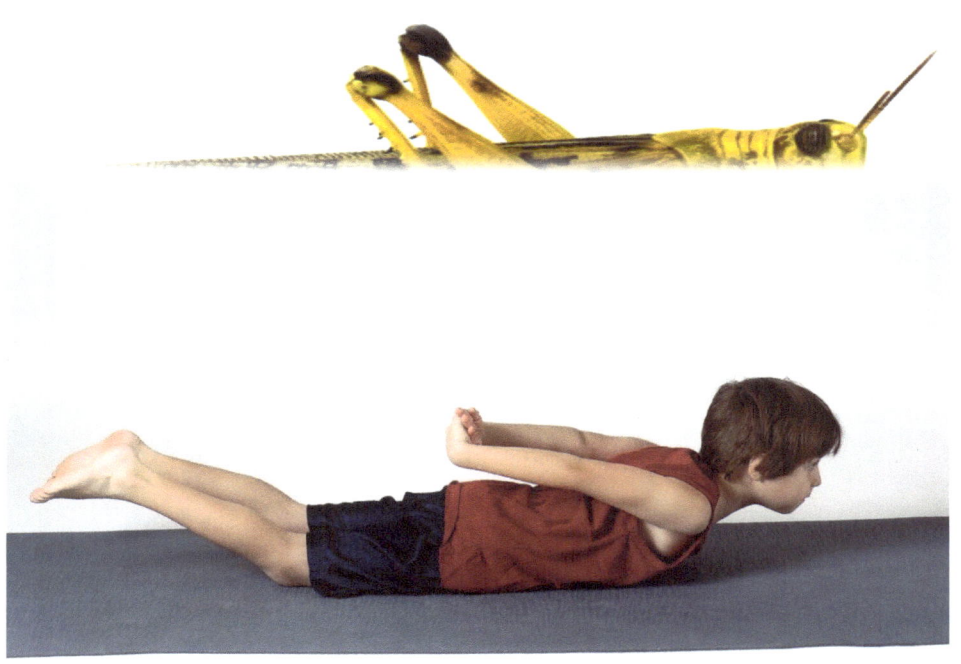

Locust

Salabhasana variation
(Sha-la-BAHS-anna)

Lay on your belly face down with your big toes touching.
Clasp your arms behind you, arch your back.
Lift your heart and look strait ahead.
If you can, lift up your feet.

 Strengthens lower back & core, reduces fatigue.

"Did you know that Locusts and Grasshoppers
are closely related and have similar habits?
Locusts "sing" by rubbing their rear feet and wing together.
Try singing softly or rubbing your back feet and legs together"

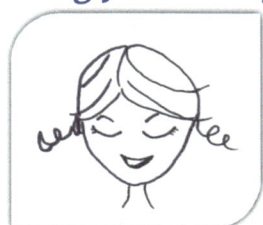

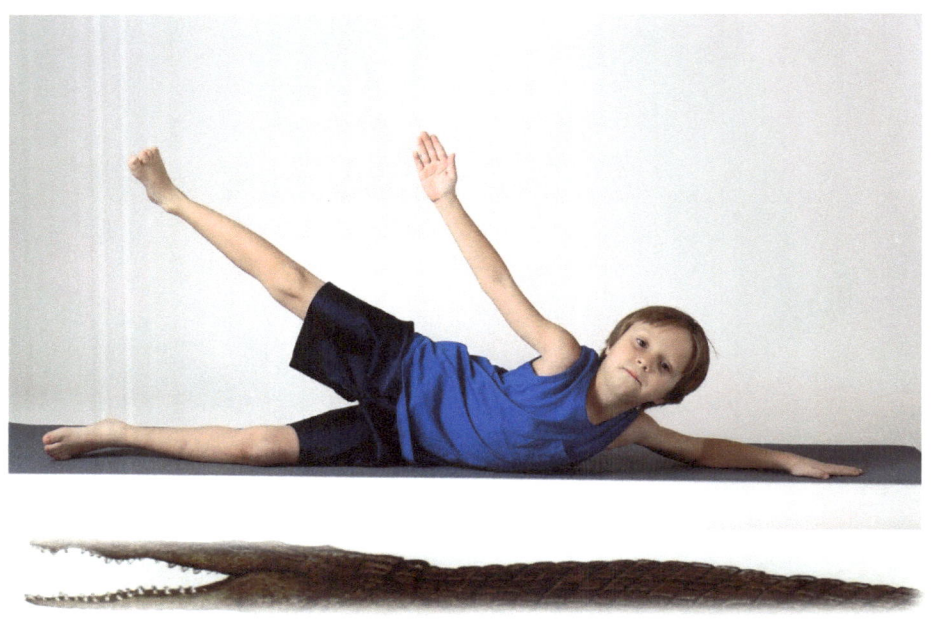

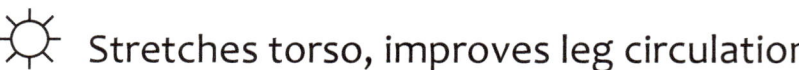

Crocodile

Anantasana variation

(A-nant-AWS-ah-nuh)

Laying on 1 side, support your head with 1 arm.
Raise your other arm up strait up to the clouds.
Lift 1 leg up and gently feel a stretch.
Hold your foot, if you can.
Repeat on opposite side.

☼ Stretches torso, improves leg circulation.

"Try snapping your Crocodile mouth closed by sending your leg back down.
Careful not to snap down too hard!
Can you try snapping down really sllloooowwwwwlllyyy?
Now try this - Breathe in (INHALE) and raise your leg...
breathe out (EXHALE) and lower your leg."

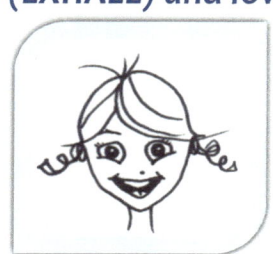

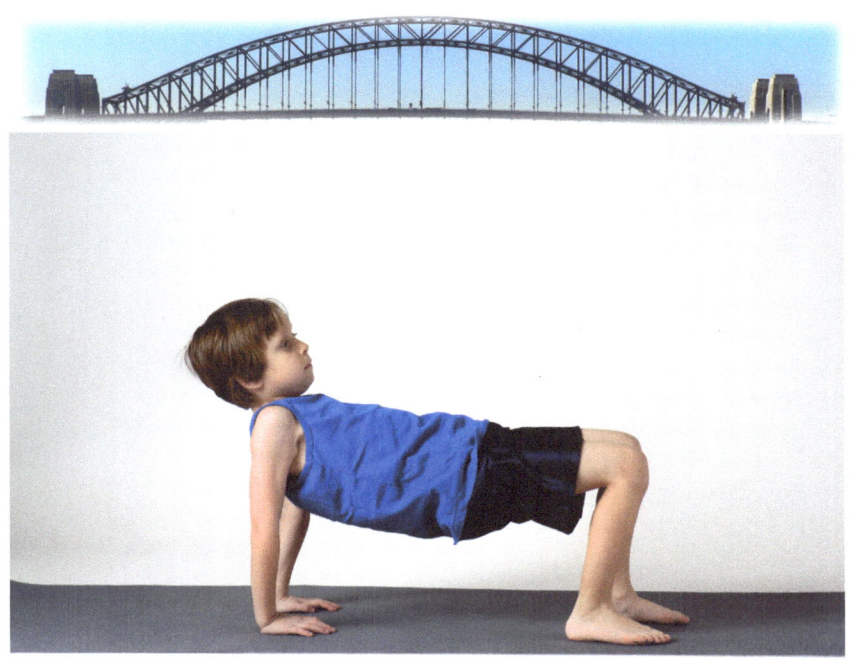

Bridge

Purvottanasana variation
(PUR-voh-tun-AHS-uh-nuh)

Starting seated, bend your knees and walk your feet forward.
Make train tracks with your feet at the front of the mat.
Straighten your arms and lift your belly.
Point your hands in the direction of your feet.
Lift your hips towards the clouds, making a bridge.

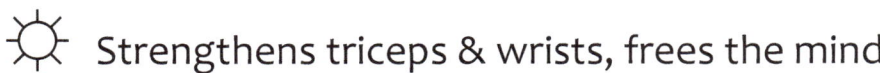 Strengthens triceps & wrists, frees the mind.

*"Imagine all the different vehicles that will pass under your bridge...
they are all different shapes and sizes.
Maybe you need to raise or lower your bridge
for the different sizes of trucks and cars."*

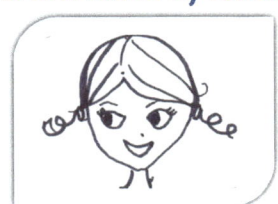

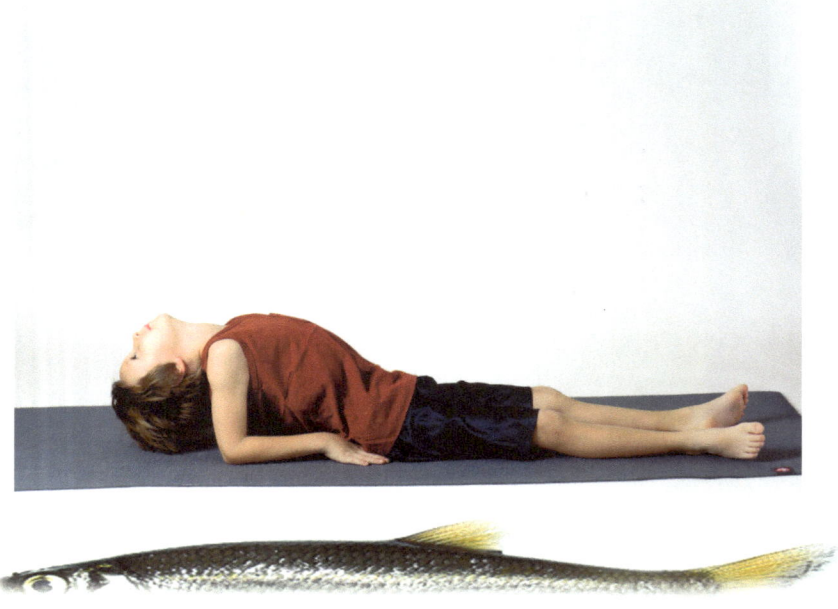

Fish

Matsyasana variation
(mot-see-AHS-anna)

Lay on your back.
Lean on your elbows propped up behind you.
Slide your hands under your bottom.
Flex your feet. Lift your heart to the clouds.
Open your mouth and let your head hang back.

 Provides extra oxygen into the lungs, opens heart.

"Swimming is so much fun. Fish breathe underwater using gills.
Take a deep breath in through your nose (INHALE) using your belly,
and then breathe out through your nose (EXHALE).
Feel your belly and your sides breathing in and out, up and down.
Use your breath to pretend that you have gills too!"

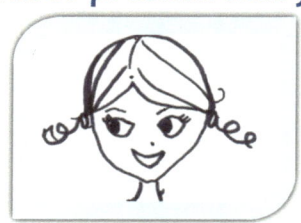

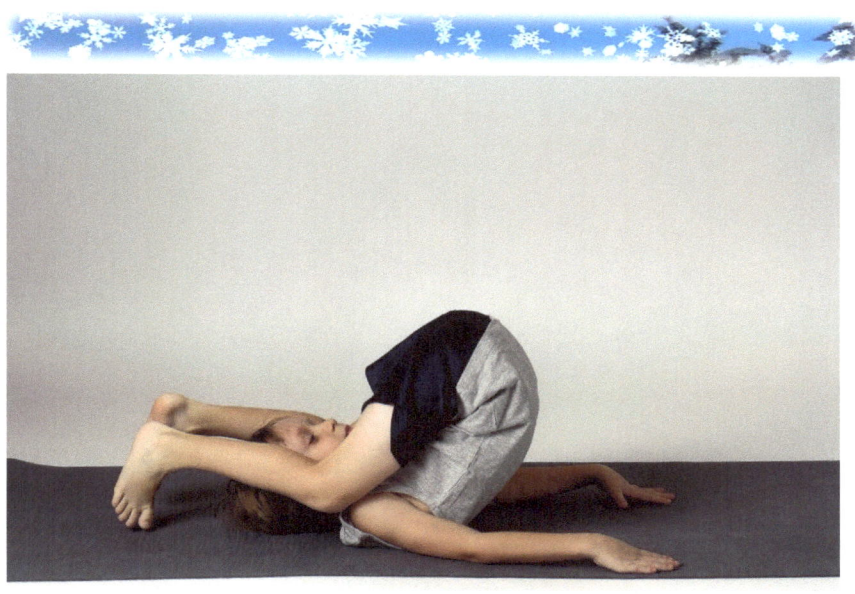

Snowplow

Halasana / Plough pose variation
(Hah-LAHS-uh-nuh)

Lay down on your mat and gaze at the sky.
Extend and press your arms to the mat.
Bring your legs up and lift your hips over your shoulders.
Roll your legs behind you,
touching your feet to the floor behind your head.

☼ Leg flexibility, stimulates multiple organs.

"As you roll backward, imagine you are a Snowplow scooping up snow!
Now hold the snow in your plow and breathe.
Using your belly, Breathe in (INHALE)
and breathe out (EXHALE) as you pause here for a moment.
Now round your back and come down. Good job!"

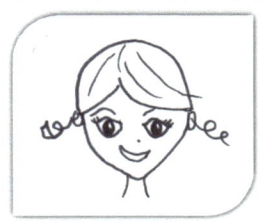

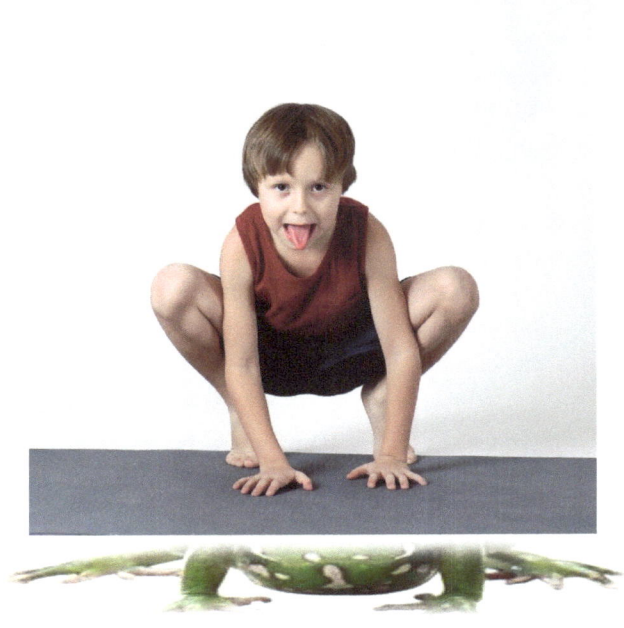

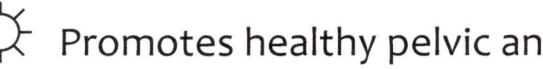

Frog

Malasana variation

(Mah-LAHS-anna)

**Stand at center of mat,
Squat down with your feet hip width apart.
Turn your toes out slightly.
Knees aligned over ankles.
Hands pressed into the ground in front.**

☼ Promotes healthy pelvic and hip joints.

*"Frogs eat insects! Wow!! When a Frog catches an insect,
it throws its tongue out to catch it!
Every different species of Frog has their own look.
They come in so many colors and patterns!"*

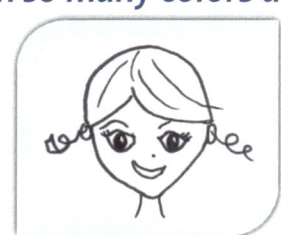

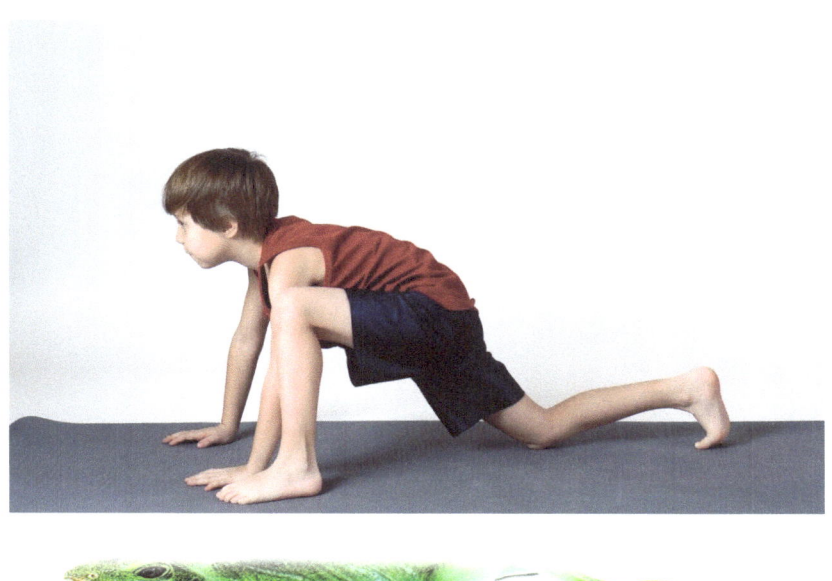

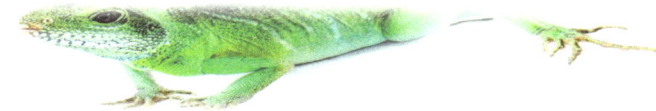

Lizard

Utthan Pristhasana variation
(OOT-ahn preesth- AHS – anna)

Start in the center of your mat. Step and lunge 1 foot forward
Now place your elbows and forearms down and strait out in front.
Relax your hips and settle them down.
Extend your heart forward, looking strait ahead.
Repeat on other side.

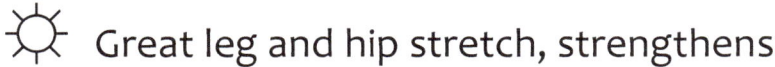 Great leg and hip stretch, strengthens.

"Lizards smell by licking the air just like snakes do!
Lizards are really good climbers and they love the hot sun!
Their camouflage and speed can make them tricky to spot.
Imagine you are a lizard getting ready to climb a rock in the hot sun."

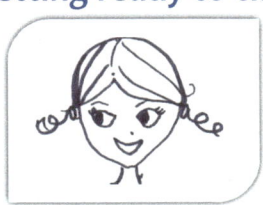

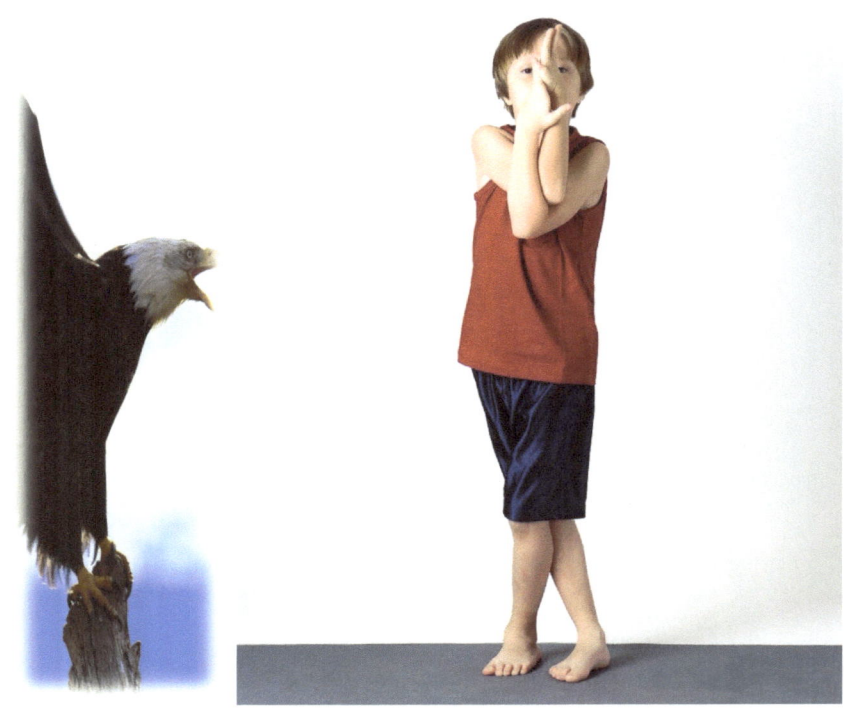

Eagle

Garudasana
(Gah-rue-DAHS-anna)

Stand in the middle of your mat.
Cross 1 leg over the other and bend your knees slightly.
Fold 1 arm under the other and wrap them together like a spiral.
Repeat spiraling opposite arm and leg.

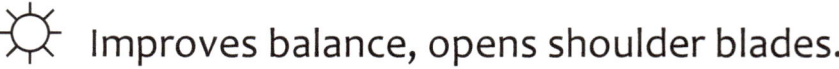 Improves balance, opens shoulder blades.

"Eagles are large and powerful. Their wings can span almost 8 feet!
Thinking of an Eagle might remind us to be courageous
and confident!
Believe in yourself. You are about to take flight!!!"

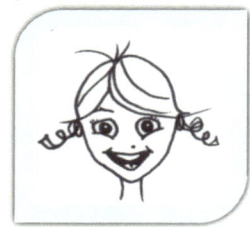

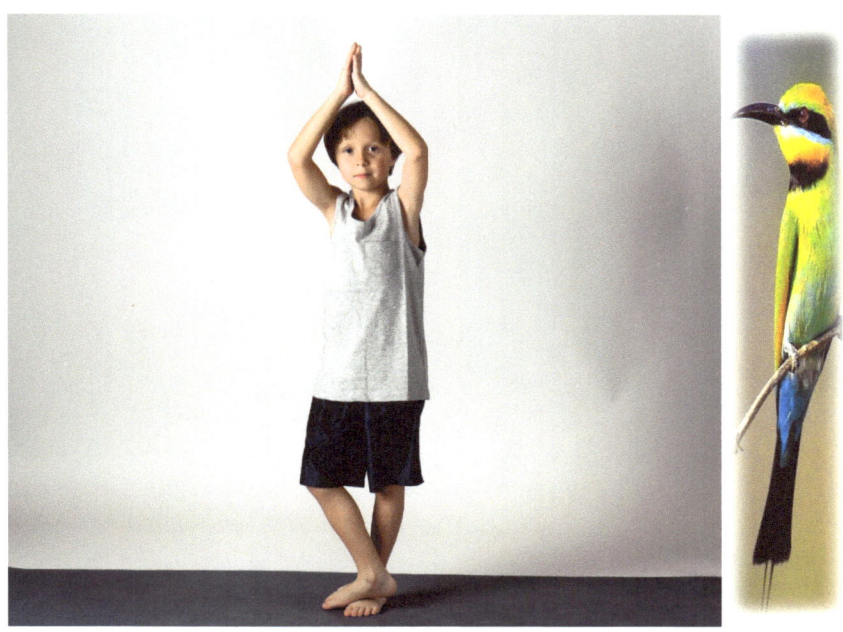

Bird

Svarga Dvidasana / Bird of Paradise variation / Tree
(Svar-gah dwee-JAHS-un-nuh)

**Stand strait and tall.
Feel your feet grounded into the floor
as if you are the planted in the ground like the root of a tree.
Bring your heel onto the top of your opposite foot.
Extend hands at Namaste up strait and tall.
Repeat using opposite foot.**

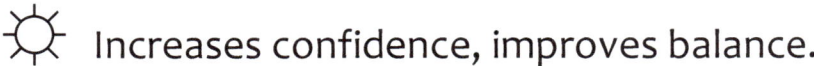 Increases confidence, improves balance.

*"What kind of bird are you?
A tropical colorful Bird? These Birds can sing songs!
Or maybe you are a hummingbird?
Let's make a humming sound together like hummingbirds."*

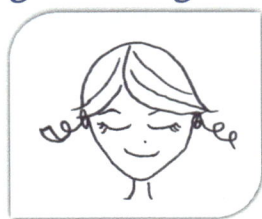

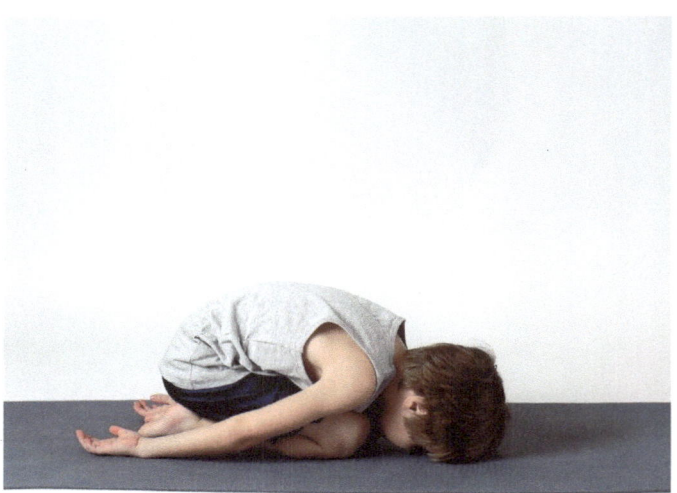

Quiet Mouse
Balasana / Child's Pose
(Bal-AHS-anna)

**Kneel down and lean over knees.
Rest your forehead gently on the mat.
Arms at sides, palms facing up.**

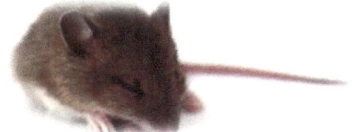 Aids circulation, calms, encourages good breathing.

*"Mice are much like humans in how their bodies and minds work.
Some people believe that mice can quietly communicate
telepathically with each other!!
Isn't that cool!?
They are also talented with swimming and climbing.
Right now, let's see what a Quiet Mouse you can be."*

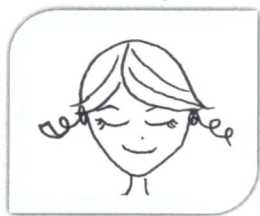

Sequence III

Kids Yoga
Suzie Cues

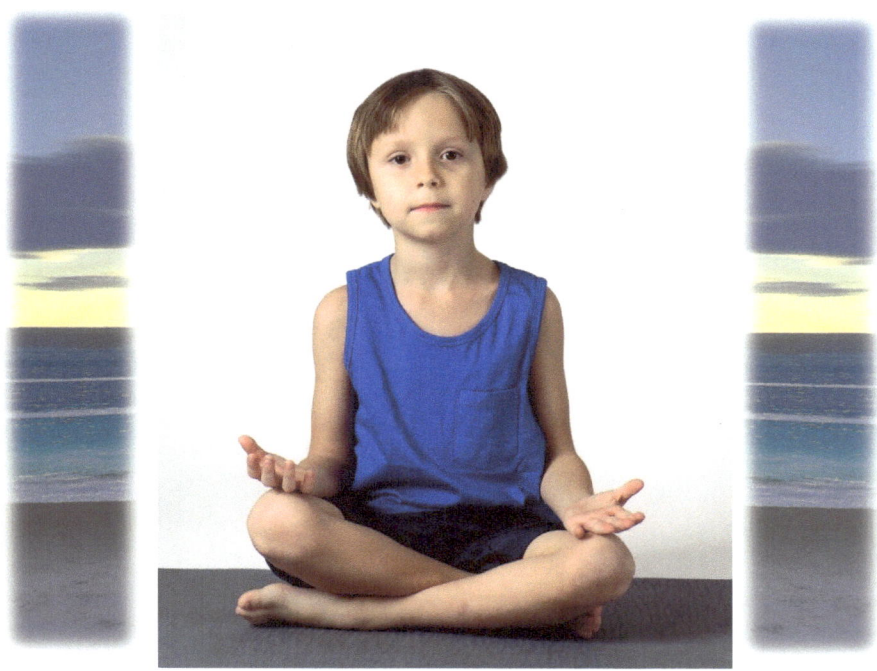

Easy Pose

Sukhasana variation
(Sookas-ana)

Sit like a pretzel.
Plant our tails into the ground. Sit up strait and tall.
Place your hands on your knees, palms facing up or down.

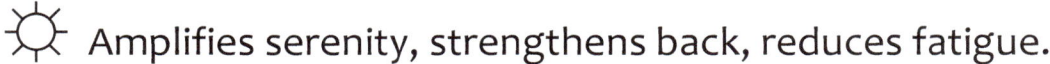 Amplifies serenity, strengthens back, reduces fatigue.

"Pretend you are a puppet on a string being pulled upward
from the very top of your head.
Gently close your eyes and enjoy this still and easy moment.
Sukha also translates to comfortable, happy, or joyful.
Try and feel what all those words feel like."

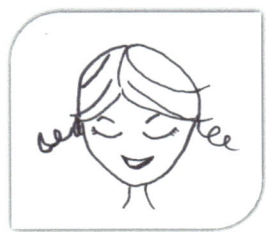

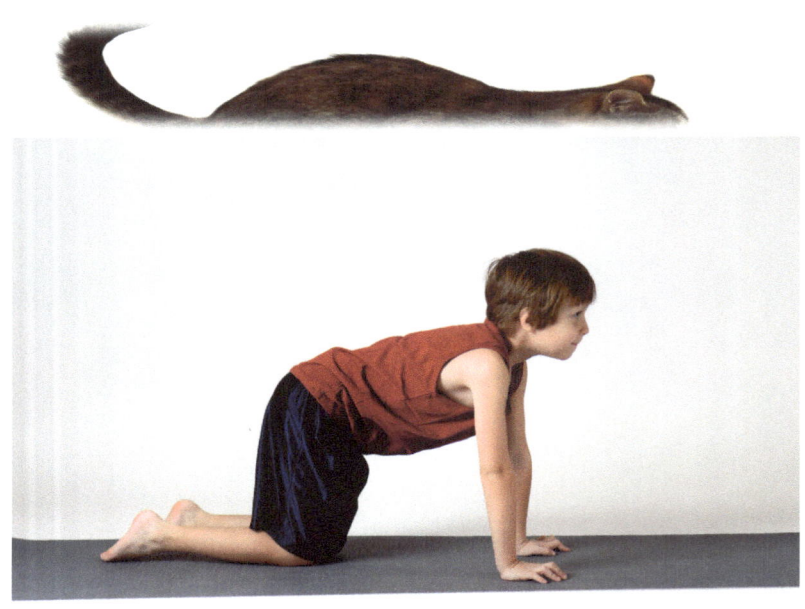

Cat

Marjaryasana variation
(mahr-jahr-ee-AHS-uh-nuh)

Kneel with your feet planted down firmly.
Hi Five the floor in front of you.
Straighten your arms, elbows bent slightly.
<u>Round</u> your back.
Look strait and down.

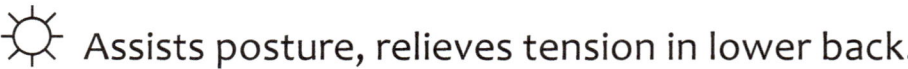 Assists posture, relieves tension in lower back.

"Meeeeooooowww!!
What color is your fur? What kind of cat are you?
Are you a quiet sneaky cat or a loud Halloween cat?
As you round your back, make the shape of an umbrella.
You can also combine Cat pose with Cow pose-
Inhale and Mooooo!! Exhale and Meowwww!!!

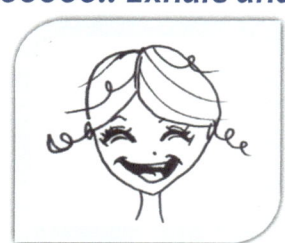

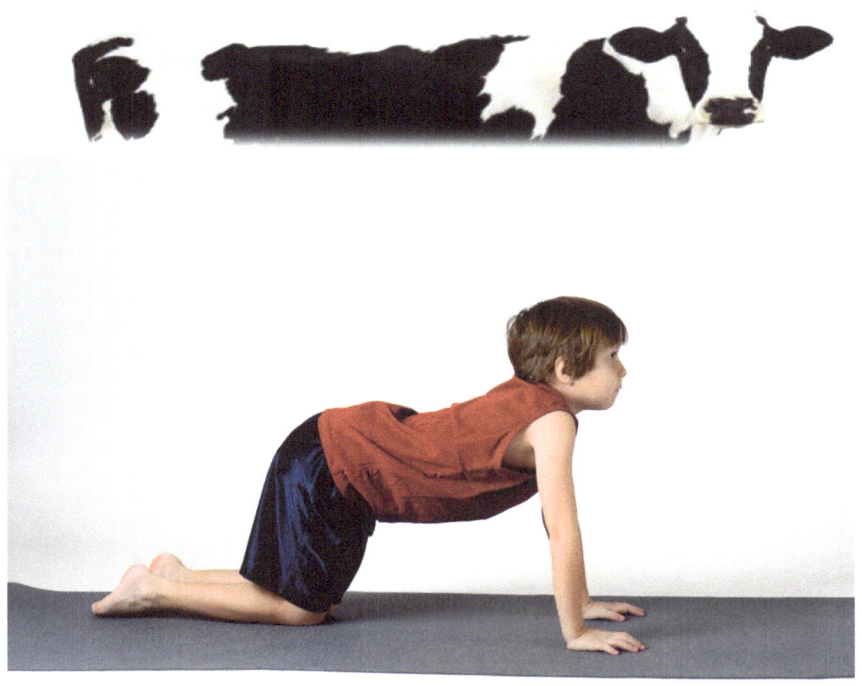

Cow

Bitilasana variation
(Bi- til-ahs- anna)

While kneeling, Hi Five the floor.
Lift your tail upward and lift your heart.
<u>Arch</u> your back.
Look strait ahead.

 Improves posture, excellent stretch, relieves pain.

"Moooo!! Did you know that Cows sometimes sleep while standing??
And did you know that every day Cows drink about a bathtub full of water??
If you haven't already tried it, you can combine Cow pose with Cat pose!
Inhale and Mooooo like a Cow!!! Exhale and Meeewooooww!!

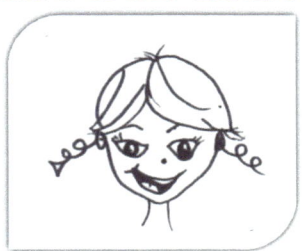

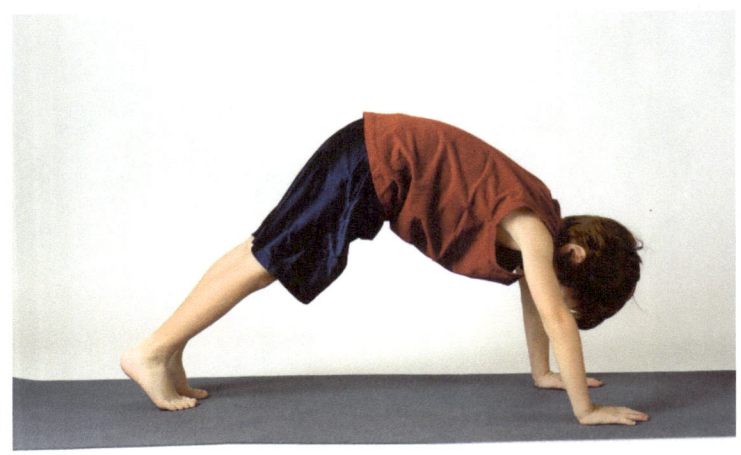

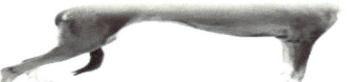

Downward Facing Dog

Adho Mukha Svanasana variation
(AH-doh MOO-kah -shvah-Nahs-anna)

Hi Five the floor beneath your shoulders.
Walk your feet back into train tracks in line with your hands.
Lift up your bottom, as if there was a
string pulling your hips upward.
Look toward your belly button.
Press your heels down.
Let your head hang and look toward your belly.

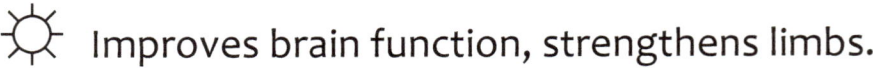 Improves brain function, strengthens limbs.

"Can you lift your leg to make a wagging tail?
Dogs are great companions and cuddly friends, and they love to give love!
What sounds do dogs make?
What expressions do they make?
They are a lot like us, don't you think?"

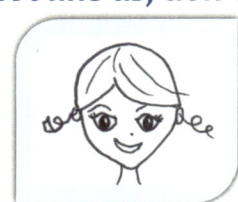

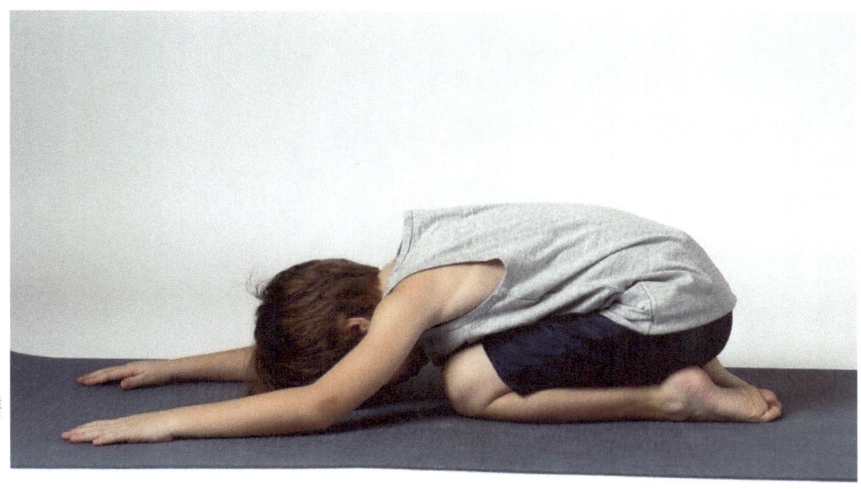

Stretching Puppy

Uttana Shishosana / Extended Puppy variation
(Ooo-tana Shish-os-anna)

**Start on all 4s, walk hands forward.
High five the floor with both hands.
Keep knees where they are. Pull your hips back.
Stretch forward and then drop your chest down.
Let your forehead touch the mat.
Relax your neck and feel the stretch.**

☼ Improves flexibility, stretches spine & shoulders.

*"Most of a Puppy's life is spent sleeping and eating
... sounds like a Puppy's life is pretty awesome and relaxing!!
They grow as they sleep and have a strong sense
of touch, so they need A LOT of good cuddles!
Stretch and take a rest here just like a sweet little Puppy!"*

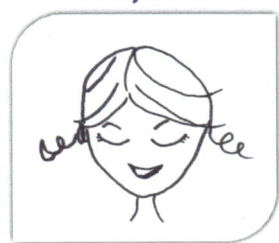

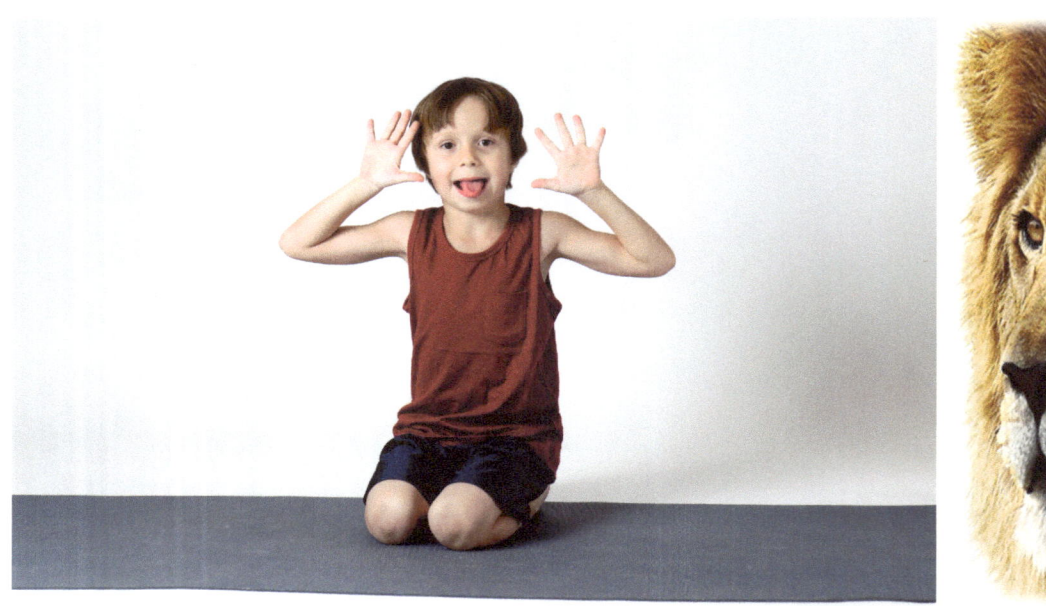

Lion

Simhasana variation
(Sim-HAHS-anna)

**Kneel on the floor. Cross you back ankles.
Rest palms on knees
and then fan out your hands next to your face on either side.**

☼ Stimulates nerves, improves circulation, makes you happy!

*"Open your eyes and mouth wide!
Stretch your tongue, and exhale using the Haaahh sound to make your ROAR!!
Did you know that Lions are really big cats??
Baby Lions are called cubs.
The roar of a Lion can be heard from 5 miles away!
That is loud!*

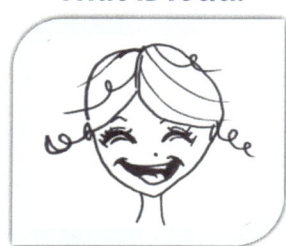

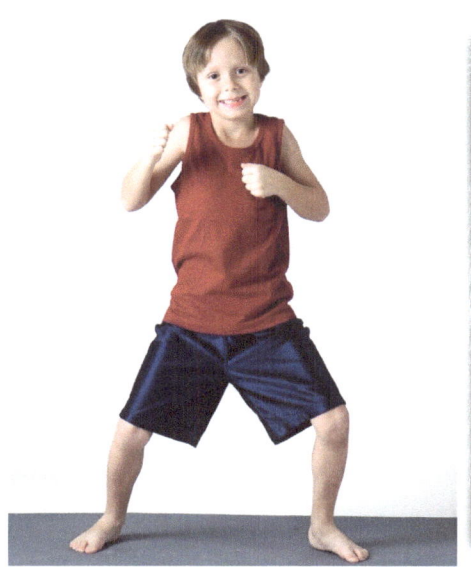
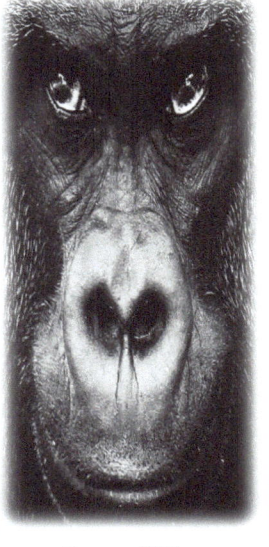
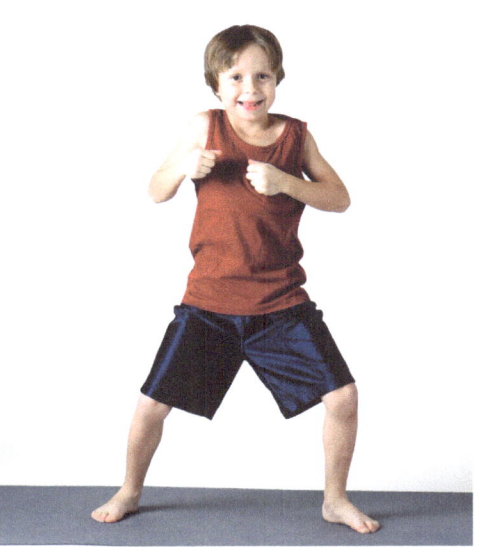

Gorilla

Prasarita Padottanasana / Standing forward bend variation
(Pra-sa-REE-tah pah-doh-tahn-AHS-anna)

Take a wide stance.
Bend knees over ankles
Make your spine tall and pound your chest like a Gorilla!

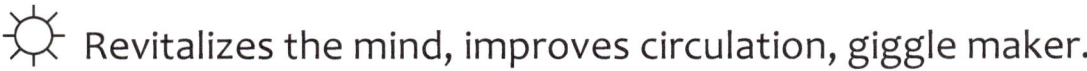 Revitalizes the mind, improves circulation, giggle maker.

"Did you know that Gorillas have fingerprints just like you and me??
AND they also have nose prints!
They eat a lot of fruit and they love bamboo!
Breathe into your Gorilla belly (INHALE)
and enjoy a loud Gorilla roar as you breathe out (EXHALE)"

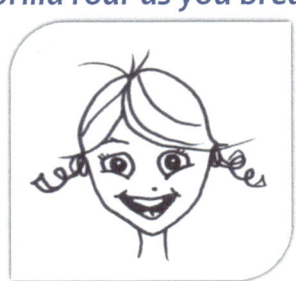

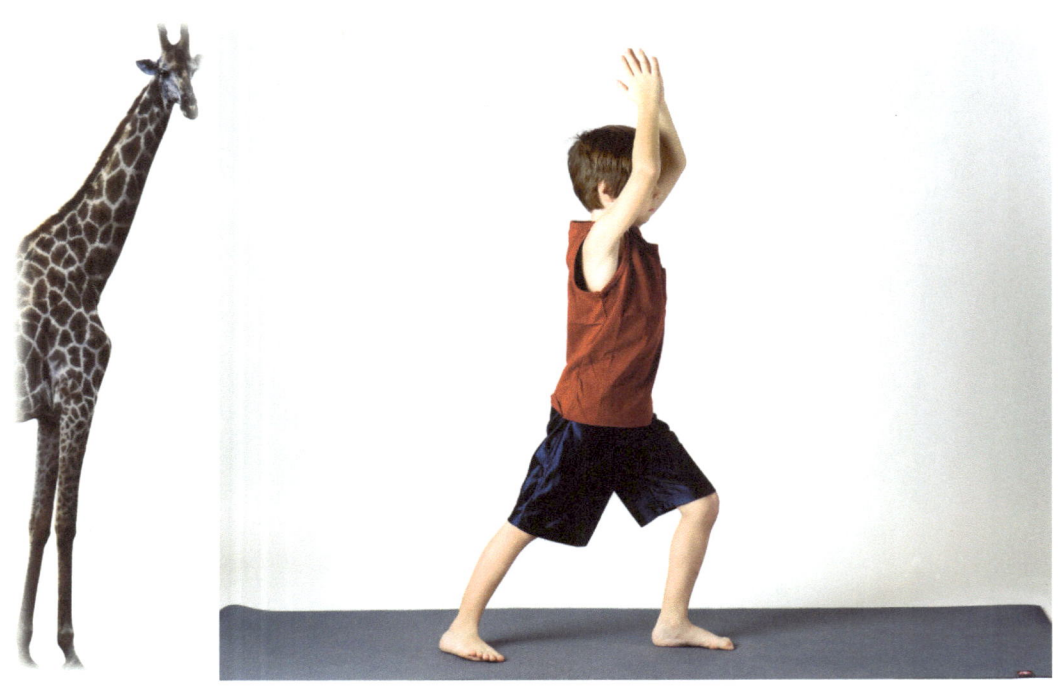

Giraffe

Virabhadrasana / Warrior I variation
(Veer-ah-bah-DRAHS-anna)

**Stand in the center of your mat.
Step 1 foot forward, knee above the ankle.
Angle back leg.
Raise arms overhead. Shoulders relaxed away from ears.
Press palms together making a tall giraffe neck.
Repeat the pose on the opposite side.**

 Develops balance, improves respiration, energizes.

*"Giraffes are the tallest land animals!
Their legs alone are 6 feet tall, and the baby calves are 6 feet tall at birth!
How tall can you stretch??"*

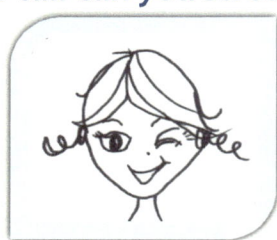

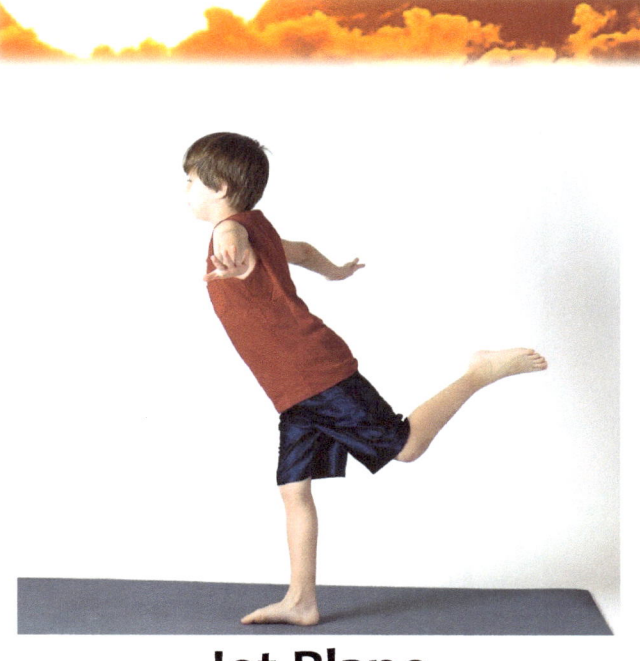

Jet Plane

Virabhadrasana III / Warrior III varitation
(Veer-ah-bah-DRAHS-anna)

Standing at center of mat strait and tall.
Plant both feet firmly into the ground.
Balancing on 1 foot, lift the other foot strait back
like the tail of a jet plane.
Make the Jet's wings extending both arms out. Lean forward.
Repeat, balancing on other foot.

 Tones body, improves concentration, strengthens.

*"Jets are super-fast and fly much faster and higher than an airplane.
The powerful noise a jet makes is from the shockwaves it makes in the air.
What does your jet plane sound like? Vvvrrrrmmmmmmmm!!!!!"*

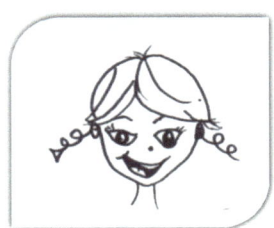

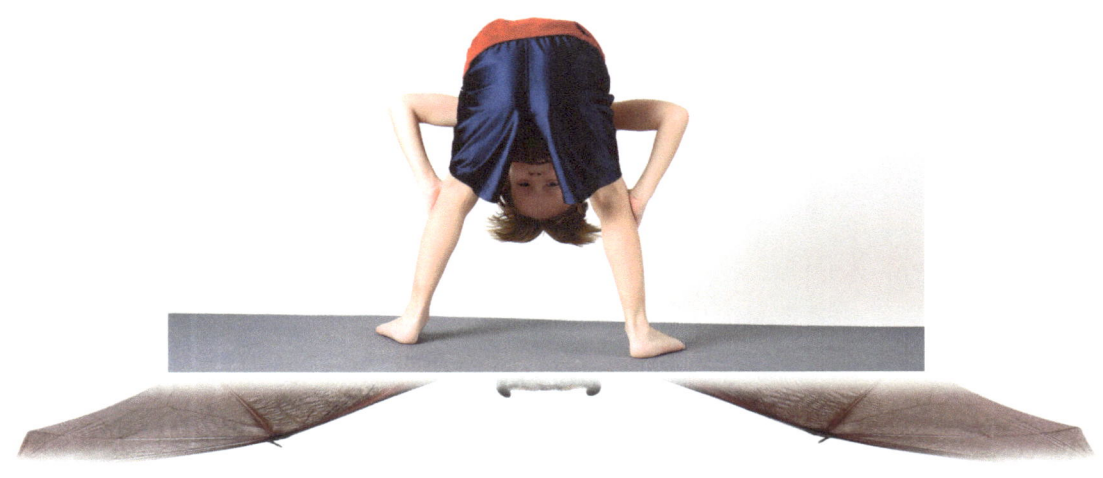

Vampire Bat

Prasarita Padottanasana / Wide-legged forward bend variation
(Pra-sa-REE-tah Pah-doh-tahn-AHS-anna)

Turn your body around and face the other way.
Take a wide stance and make train tracks with your feet.
Bend forward.
Place hands on the front of your thighs to create bat wings.
Look through your legs.

 Tones abdominals, strengthens inner legs & spine.

"Smile- and let's see those Vampire fangs!!
SO much fun!! What color are your fangs? Red? Purple?
Take a moment here to breathe.
How do you feel when you hang your head and breathe?
Did you know that bats can sleep upside down??!!!"

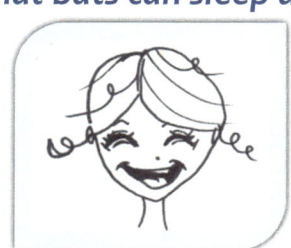

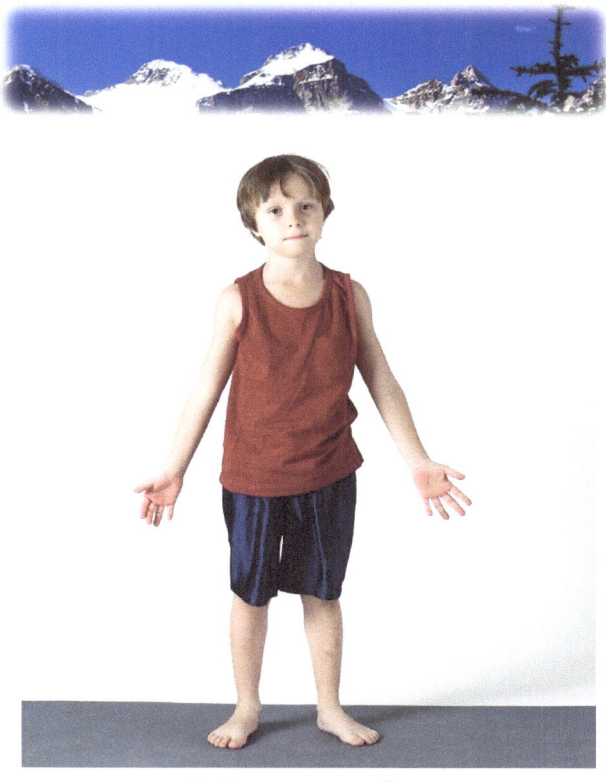

Mountain

Tasadana variation

(Tah-DAHS-anna)

Stand in center of mat. Standing tall with eyes closed (or open). Hands open palms facing forward.

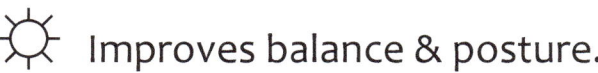 Improves balance & posture.

"Have you ever been Mountain climbing?
A Mountain inspires us to stand firmly on our own two feet.
The world's tallest Mountain is Mount Everest, and it continues to grow!
It's so quiet and peaceful at the top of a Mountain.
How quiet and peaceful do you feel right now?"

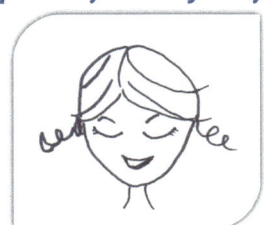

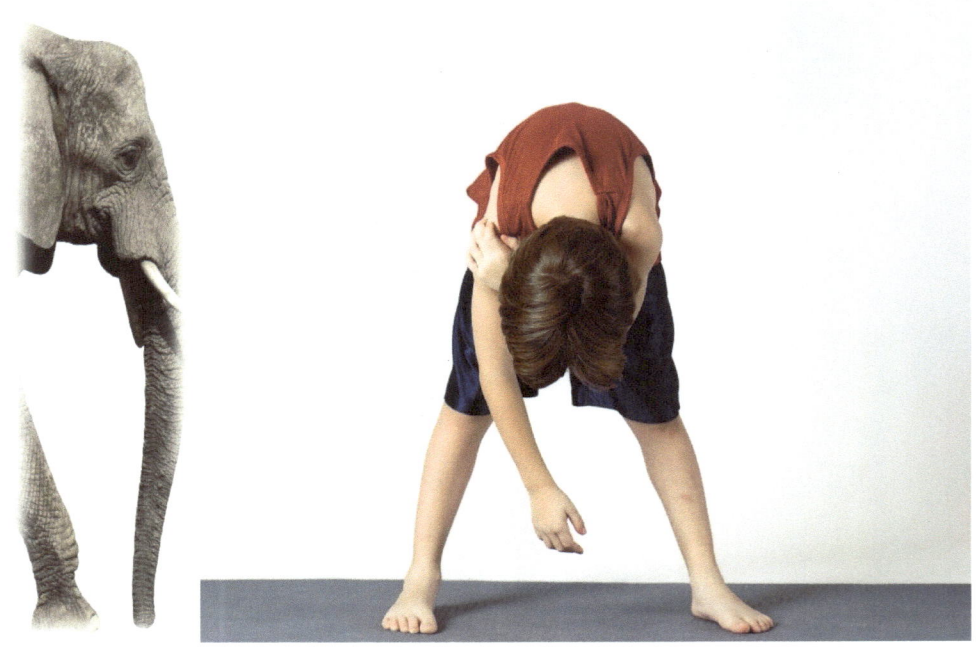

Elephant

Uttanasana variation
(OOT-tan-AHS-ahna)

**Make train tracks with your feet in standing position.
Forward bend and let your upper body
and head hang soft and heavy.
Grab your elbows with your hands
and then let 1 arm hand down long
like the trunk of an elephant.**

☼ Calms the brain, stretches legs & hips.

*"Stomp your legs back and forth like a huge heavy elephant!
Can you guzzle up some water with your trunk like an elephant??
Let's sip, guzzle, and spray our friends with the water!"*

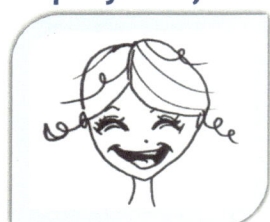

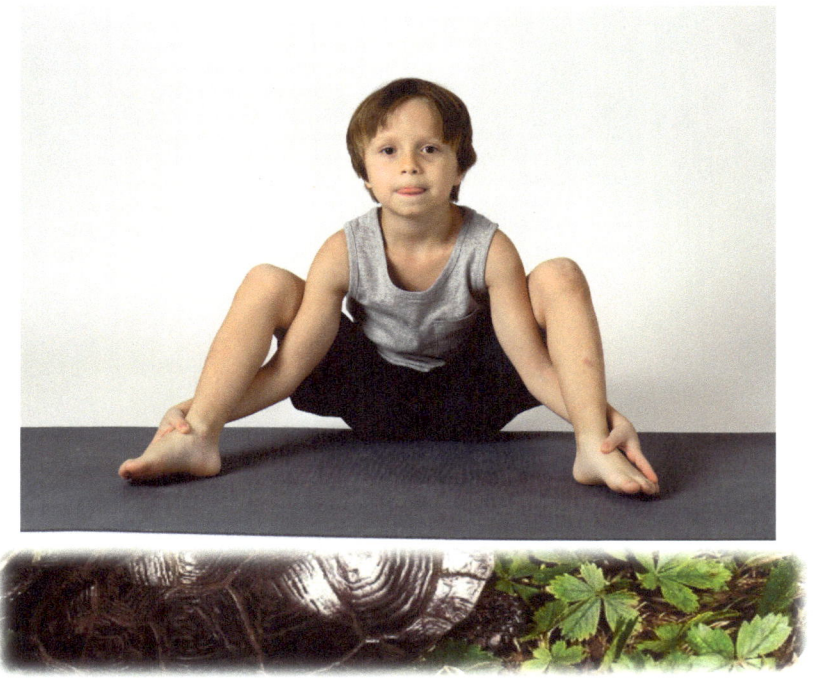

Turtle

Kurmasana variation
(Kur-MAHS-anna)

Sit legs out wide.
Bend knees slightly.
Slip hands beneath your knees under your legs.
Keep a strait back, and look forward.

☀ Releases tightness in the back, lengthens back.

"Turtles have been on our planet for more than 200 million years
– Probably because the unique hard shells protect them!
This shell gives them a place to hide for safety!
Relax into the pose and name a place that you feel safe.
You can say it silently to yourself or share it out loud."

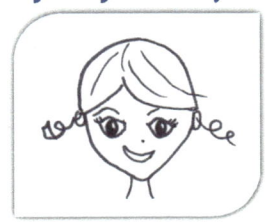

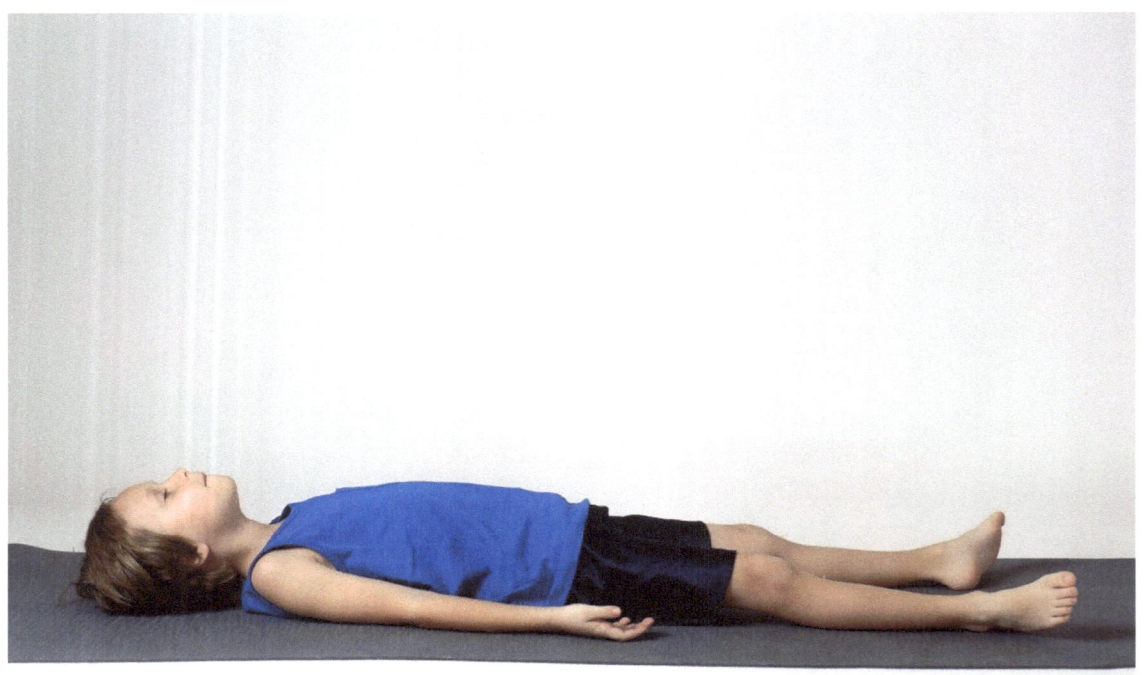

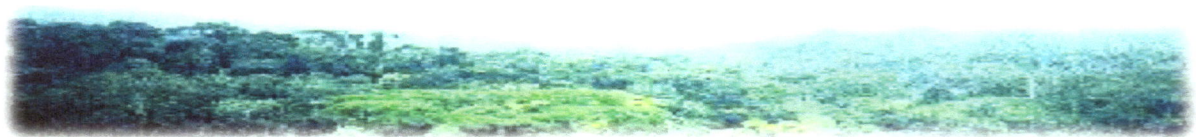

A Quiet Ride in the Rainforest

Savasana variation
(Shah-VAHS-anna)

**In a dim or quiet room,
Lay down with your arms at your sides.
Gently close your eyes.
Palms facing toward the clouds.
Soften and relax your body. Relax your face.
Breathe.
Feel the rhythm of your breathing.
Listen to the guided meditation.**

 Rejuvenates while connecting body & mind.

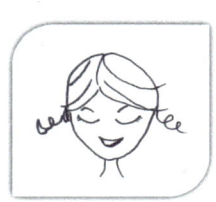

"Imagine you are laying on a bed of soft green leaves in the rainforest.
Notice the way the leaves feel soft and comfortable beneath you.
Can you imagine more details about your bed of leaves?
What color is it? How does the air around you feel and smell?
It can look or feel any way you choose.

Without moving, imagine the bed of leaves lifting you up on a gentle ride,
guiding you through the Rainforest.
You feel light as air as you are lifted... drifting slowly.
Feel the warm sun on your face
and a soft watery mist in the air, as if it has just rained.

As you travel on your gentle ride,
listen to the sounds of the rainforest and the animals that live here.
As you look around, you can see these animals,
they are happily playing and moving through the Rainforest.
Birds, Frogs, Snakes, Lizards, Monkeys,..
You hear the animals too, making their sounds near and far in the distance.

As you are listening, you also hear a stream of moving water.
Your bed of leaves softly stops moving and rests you down beside it.
What color is the water? Do you stop to dip your feet inside?
Maybe there is a small waterfall you can feel with your hands.
As you sit beside the water,
look up at the trees that fill the space around you.
Notice the blue sky and soft white clouds beyond the trees.

Imagine a beautiful butterfly landing softly on your belly.
(optional: place a toy or paper butterfly on each child's belly)
As you breathe, you can watch the butterfly move gently
up and down with your breath.
As you breathe in, the butterfly lifts...
As you breathe out, the butterfly lowers.
Enjoy a quiet moment and a couple rounds of breathing

When you feel like it..., gently open your eyes."

A Note From the Author

"When I was 5 years old, my mother always told me that happiness was the key to life.

When I went to school, they asked me what I wanted to be when I grew up. I wrote down 'happy'.

They told me I didn't understand the assignment, and I told them they didn't understand life."

-John Lennon

I started practicing yoga and mindfulness regularly,
without the expectation of change.
I went through the postures
without comprehending how to connect my breath
or how to be in the moment with myself.
Yoga slowly pushed me to be aware of myself not only physically,
but also in my heart and mind.
My muscles toned, headaches diminished,
I slept better, I was self-aware,
I appreciated more, and I felt more present.
I felt myself surrender.
Not surrender to life, but surrender to myself.
I felt myself become lighter and alive with possibility.
Life became less messy as I became more present.

Namaste,

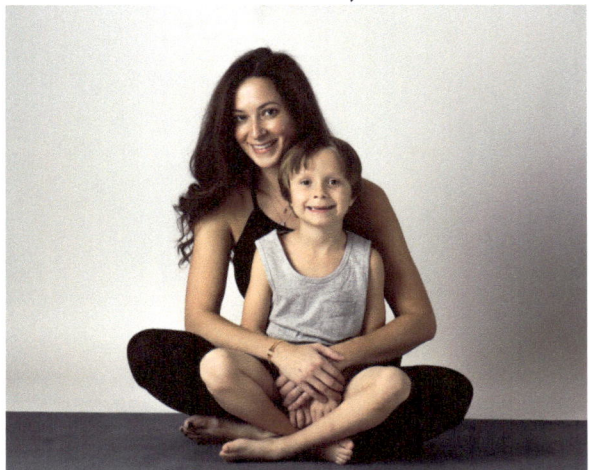

Rita Rainieri-Polak, RCYT

@MoveChillYoga

Notes

Notes

www.ingramcontent.com/pod-product-compliance
Lightning Source LLC
Chambersburg PA
CBHW040306010626
45792CB00025B/1132